C000186986

WELL
DONE
ME

WELL DONE ME

A MEMOIR

CORDELIA FELDMAN

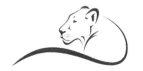

First published 2021 by Dandelion Digital,
an imprint of Paper Lion Ltd
13 Grayham Road, New Malden, Surrey, KT3 5HR, UK
www.paperlionltd.com
info@paperlionltd.com

Text copyright © Cordelia Feldman 2021

Cordelia Feldman has asserted her rights under the
Copyright, Designs and Patents Act 1988,
to be identified as Author of this work.

All rights reserved. No part of this work may be reproduced or
recorded without the permission of the publisher, in writing.

A catalogue record for this book is available from the British Library

ISBN
Paperback: 978-1-908706-41-6
eBook: 978-1-908706-42-3

Design: cover by Two Associates, interior by seagulls.net

This book is dedicated to
Mum, Dad, Alexander and Spitfire

Flash Start

For much of my life, I haven't been present. Years of medication for my bipolar disorder, plus the illness itself, mixed with large quantities of leisure drugs in my late teens and early twenties, and buckets of alcohol throughout my whole adult life, has left my memory hazy. It's only now I've been clean and sober for almost five years that I feel present in my life. The mist has vanished and a clarity of thought has arrived. I know what I'm doing and what I've done.

So, this is a book about becoming present in life: with all the challenges that entails. It's a tale of recovery, to an extent, but also one of learning to live in the moment – however terrifying. For it's only in the moment that we're truly alive. There will be laughter along the way, and tears, great suffering and greater joy.

I suffer from bipolar 1 disorder and secondary breast cancer, but this book is about more than that. It's about finding hope in a hopeless place and wonder in the everyday. It's about the ability of the human spirit to regenerate, and finding hidden strengths within yourself. Along the way you'll meet a host of characters: my parents, friends, cat, dogs and boyfriends.

This book is not meant to take the place of medical treatment or talking therapies. I'm an expert by experience on my own illnesses, but I don't make any claim to know the answers. You'll find hints and tips for dealing with depression and hypomania, chemotherapy and radiotherapy. These are all my own views and not sanctioned by any medical practitioners. I hope you enjoy the book.

Introduction

I'm sitting up in bed at my parental home, writing this on Mum's computer. At the moment I spend about four days per week here, and three days at my flat. This house, where I spent the first thirty years of my life, is in Radlett in leafy Hertfordshire, just on the edge of the green belt. My cat Spitfire, also known as the Fluffy Monster, or more recently, Precious Angel Fluffball, lives here as I am too ill to look after him.

It's 2021, and my life looks like this: personal training once a week; two regular dog-walking clients, Pilates once a week, barre Pilates twice a week. No actual job since being sacked from my dream one at a new bookshop in Radlett. Before that I worked part-time at an authors' and actors' agency for nigh on fifteen years. Seb, the love of my life, split up with me at the end of March five years ago. We'd been together on and off over a period of eleven years. More, no doubt much more, to come on Seb later. My new man is called Film Chap. We will meet him soon.

This is the house where *A Clockwork Orange* was filmed. Designed by Richard Rogers and Norman Foster, it was hailed as a modernist masterpiece and Stanley Kubrick saw it whilst scouting for locations for the film and fell in love with it. It's the house of the writer who is injured and whose wife is raped by Alex and the Droogs. Spitfire has just turned seven and a half. My brother lives in Haifa in Israel. The panther is here now.

"What's the point of you writing a memoir?" the panther asks, gazing at me with amber eyes. "Who do you think is going to want to read about your life? You don't do anything or …"

"It's going to be a book about living with mental illness, living with cancer, living in recovery from addiction," I say. "People say I'm brave and inspirational and …"

"But you're not," the panther says. "You're fat, unemployed and unemployable as far as I can tell, lazy …"

"If I write it, and it's good, they will read it," I say, feeling unsure about this. The panther returns to grooming his flank with his sandpaper tongue. I stroke the soft back of his neck. He rests his enormous head on my shoulder. His breath smells of rotting meat.

I used to suffer with writer's block until I completed a National Novel Writing Month (NaNoWriMo) challenge, set up by a group of techies in San Francisco. It's an output challenge, the aim is to write fifty thousand words of a new novel in a month. That first November I wrote sixty thousand words. Ever since then, I haven't had a problem with writer's block. Also: for the last few years I've been writing a blog. First it was a dating after breast cancer surgery one called *Scars, Tears and Training Bras,* and now it's one about exercise and my life, my bipolar disorder and secondary breast cancer called *The Rapid Cyclist*. So, I write every day. And people read my writing every day. As to whether it's any good or not, I try not to worry about that. I've just published my first novel "*In Bloom*" to rave reviews. It's doing really well.

This, though: this has to be good or no one will publish it. And no one will read it. And ever since a whole army of publishers rejected my first novel some thirteen years ago, I've been putting off starting another major project due to the fear of writing hundreds and thousands of words that no one will read. But in recent times I have been reading a lot of memoirs: Amy Liptrot's brilliant *The*

Outrun about her recovery from alcoholism, A A Gill's *Pour Me* about overcoming alcoholism and Bryony Gordon's *Mad Girl* about her obsessive-compulsive disorder. I've just read the Karl Knausgaard series which begins with '*A Death in the Family*'. There's been a thought at the back of my mind that I'm reading these memoirs for research, that perhaps a memoir rather than another novel is what I will write. And so, at last, I'm starting.

My psychiatrist Dr Joshua Stein, who I've been seeing privately for nearly twenty years, put me on Librium to stop me drinking when I went into hospital for a major cancer operation on 30th August 2016, so I've been sober for almost five years now. Part of me thought it was the drinking stopping me from doing proper writing. I no longer have that excuse: I have a clear head, space, time and writing to do. Now is the time for action. I'm almost forty-two, I wanted to publish a book by forty and managed to publish *In Bloom* just a year later.

I'm tired, so very tired. I'm on ten different medications for my breast cancer and my bipolar and other things. Let me list them:

- Latuda: lurasidone, an antipsychotic for my bipolar, as a mood stabiliser.
- Venlafaxine: a selective serotonin norepinephrine reuptake inhibitor (SNRI) or antidepressant.
- GemCarbo chemotherapy: gemcitabine and carboplatin.
- Fexofenadine: a non-drowsy antihistamine, for my allergies.
- Clonazepam: an anti-anxiety benzodiazepine to help me stay off alcohol.
- Sodium docusate: for constipation caused by the cancer drugs.
- Zolpidem: to help me sleep.
- Bisphosphonate implant: to seal my bones against cancer and to strengthen them, as osteoporosis is a common menopausal side effect.

- Colecalciferol and calcium carbonate: calcium and vitamin D supplement to go with the bisphosphonates.
- Vitamin C: to guard against colds, from which I suffer due to abnormally thickened nasal passages, the result of allergic rhinitis which I have had all my life.

The cumulative effect of all these treatments is to make me exhausted and nauseated. Plus, I do Pilates or barre or personal training on Zoom every day. I tend to sleep for up to three hours in the afternoon. This book will be written in one late morning session and one early evening session every day. I'm starting to worry about it. And my shoulder is hurting. But I must focus and write.

When he found out, in 2014, that my cancer had spread to my lungs, my oncologist gave me two years. I've already survived almost six years on top of that, so I'm living on borrowed time. All the more reason to start this book. It's going to be tough going, though, due to feeling so ill most of the time. The medical treatment described in this book is a mixture of NHS and private: NHS Breast Care Clinic; cancer diagnosis at Accident and Emergency; NHS chemotherapy; private surgery; private radiotherapy; ongoing check-up appointments with private oncologist and breast surgeon; private appointments with plastic surgeon; private psychiatrist for the last twenty years and later private psychologist; private administration of bisphosphonate and GemCarbo chemotherapy. Like various other cancer patients I know, my treatment has been a mixture of some treatments available on the NHS and others – like bisphosphonates – that at the moment are only available with health insurance.

As I write this I'm in a period of hypomania which has been going on for six weeks. Now my mood has come up, writing and life have become easier. I'm going to do two thousand words of this before turning to the blog, which I have to write and post every day without fail. One second: I must find some lemon squash. Now I don't drink alcohol I consume vast quantities of lemon squash and fizzy water, Diet Coke and coffee. It's swings and roundabouts once you're sober.

Where will this memoir start? I wonder. It could begin with my bipolar diagnosis aged twenty-four, in 2003. Or with my breast cancer diagnosis aged thirty-three. I don't have the energy to describe my unremarkable childhood, and yet I was a gifted child, so maybe that's important, growing up in a middle-class Jewish household in Radlett, Hertfordshire and attending the academic private girls' school North London Collegiate in Edgware from seven to eighteen. Or we could begin with my clubbing and ecstasy years which are covered in my first novel *In Bloom*. At the moment I'm writing my way into this, trying to find a voice.

I put on twenty-two pounds with the initial cancer treatment. Having maintained a weight of between nine and nine and a half stone for the previous nine years or so, this was a bitter blow. I didn't start to lose the weight until I stopped drinking, when it dropped off. I no longer weigh myself.

At my heaviest, when I came out of the mental hospital aged twenty-four, I weighed fourteen stone two, but I dropped five stone on a weight loss drug, Orlistat, and doing legs, bums and tums classes and lifting weights in Body Pump. Weightlifting is something I do at least once a week now, once with my trainer – I'm now too ill to do Body Pump – and it makes me feel better. I write poems about it, and maybe I will include some in this book. Lifting makes me feel strong, powerful, and it gives me the toned arms and legs I dreamt of in the past. I now have 1, 2.5, 4 and 5 kg weights at home so I can lift them whilst watching TV. Four years ago, in 2017, I wanted to train to become a Schwinn instructor and teach indoor cycling classes, as I love it so much, but I just couldn't raise my speed or resistance during periods of low mood, so I cancelled the course as my teacher said I wouldn't pass it.

A few years ago, I completed a trial run of an eight week mindfulness meditation course for bipolar sufferers with a psychologist and that's something I do twice a day: the body scan meditation, which focuses on each body part in turn. It's just over twenty minutes long and I do it before my afternoon sleep (when I have one) and in bed at night. It helps me sleep, calms me and reduces anxiety: it's a good practice for acceptance of my current situation.

G-d, writing is hard work. I have to have to have to reach two thousand words before I stop today but so much of me wants to stop right now. I'm sending text messages to friends to say I've begun writing a memoir, in the hope of, I think, encouragement, and so some people know I'm doing it, to hold me accountable. I've announced it on the blog and on Facebook. I've told my parents, brother and best friends. I have no doubt I'll end up deleting all or most of this anyway. I have to think of where to start.

"You can't stick to it," the panther says. He's lying next to me in bed, resting his head on my shoulder. "You'll give up and ..."

"No," I say, shaking my head. "No, I won't. I'll write this whole book, you'll see."

"You haven't done any proper writing for years," the panther says, turning his head to groom himself, licking his back with his rasping tongue. "You won't be able to stick to it and ..."

"I will," I say. "This isn't fiction, this is my life. I know what happens in my life. I was there."

But was I even there? For so much of my life I've been in altered states: depressed, high, drunk or drugged with morphine, alcohol, ecstasy, antidepressants and mood stabilisers. Or with the wren of anxiety paralysing me, or mania wiping my memory. The cumulative effects of years of mental illness and its drugs stop me from remembering. This is not going to be easy; I know that. But I have to start, I have to try.

It's sunny outside and the sky is blue. Mum is calling my cat, Spitfire: he has to come in before dark and it's 5.52 p.m. now. My parents are having guests for dinner. I must have a bath and write my blog. I must find Dad who will show me how to save this document and email it to myself. Mum edits it on my computer and then I make ever more complicated pencil notes on a printed copy. We're on the eighth draft now. But these are just little niggles. This is just the process of starting something new. I'm not feeling too much in the way of fear – I will complete these two thousand words in two and a half hours which isn't brilliant going but it's not terrible.

One of the reasons I started writing this four years ago is because my boyfriend in 2017, New Chap, was finishing off an MA and then he was going to start a PhD and I didn't want him to think I wasn't using my brain. I told him about my Oxford degree and my Creative Writing MA and my unpublished novel and I wanted to impress him by producing some work and by committing to a big project. He said he wanted to read it. I wanted him to be proud of me. I wanted to be proud of myself. I wanted my parents to stop nagging me about not doing anything. Since I first started writing this I've acquired a new boyfriend, Film Chap, who for once is older than me – he's forty-one and is a film director: hence his handle.

"I hope you don't think I'm trying to trap you by knitting you a scarf," I say. We're lying on my amazing, luxuriant new grey sofa from Costco at my flat.

"I'm touched you want to knit me a scarf," he says smiling, his green eyes flashing.

"It's so sweet of you – you're a lovely person."

"Thank you so much darling," I say, kissing him, feeling relieved that at last I've met someone chilled, kind and empathetic who likes

9

me. He's got great taste in yarn too: he's chosen Lion Mandala in Thunderbird which is purple, orange, yellow and turquoise. The scarf will be stunning but at sixty stitches wide it's going to take months. I'm ecstatic he wants to stick around that long.

"Would you like a cup of Earl Grey?" I ask, hauling myself off the sofa and over to the kitchen surface where the kettle, mugs, tea and teapots live.

"Perfect," he says. Putting the kettle on, I listen to its rumble and feel content. I'm just where I need to be in this moment with my man, tea and tennis: the US Open is on Amazon Prime which I now have – happy days. Roger Federer serves yet another ace to take the set 6–1.

PART ONE

Chapter 1

2013

"I can't show you the whole tumour," the doctor says, "because it's too large for the ultrasound scanner. But it's definitely breast cancer, it's a ductal carcinoma."

"Are you sure?" I ask. It just seems impossible. I'm thirty-three years old. I didn't even know you could develop breast cancer at my age.

"We're starting chemotherapy in two weeks," my breast surgeon says. She is pretty: long black hair, smart dress. "We're going to throw everything we have at it."

"Why can't you take it out?" I ask. There is an alien growing inside me. I want to get rid of it.

"The tumour is too large," she says. "We must attempt to shrink it with chemotherapy first: because it's reached the skin we'll need to remove the affected area and you simply don't have enough skin to close the hole that will make and …"

"I don't want to have chemotherapy," I say. "I don't want to lose my hair or …"

"It's the only option," she says, her dark eyes flashing. She wears knee-high black leather boots.

So, what we thought was a rash on my skin is in fact cancer. The other signs are the heat emanating from my breast, the dimpling there which is referred to as 'orange peel' skin and is the texture of a golf ball, and the inverted nipple. It appears to be inflammatory breast cancer and my breast feels hard and hot like a pizza stone.

I'm aware that this is serious. As I sit here, holding Mum's hand, I am aware that this is unusual: to have a tumour so large that it can't be removed. In all the breast cancer stories I've ever heard it's been lump removal, then chemotherapy, then radiotherapy. So now, at this first NHS team meeting with the oncologist and breast surgeon, I know that this is worse. I'm not scared of dying: years of mental illness have familiarised me with being so depressed that I've wanted to die many times. I feel relief, in fact, that I haven't got long left. What I am terrified of, however, is chemotherapy.

"She has bipolar disorder," Mum says, stroking my hand, her face etched with worry. She looks so old and tired now. "She has such a difficult life already and …"

"I don't want to have chemotherapy," I say. "I don't want to lose my hair and get fat and … aren't I too young for this?"

"We have a patient who is twenty," my surgeon says. "Chemo-therapy starts in two weeks."

I am crying. *I am crying because of the shock*, I think. I am crying because I have waited until this late stage to do something about this. Part of it is not my fault because a ductal carcinoma starts in the duct network and works outwards, so it's only in the last few weeks that my entire breast has felt hard and hot. It went from nothing to a hot mass – there's no discrete lump. This is unlike anything I've ever read or seen about breast cancer. But I have waited until the cancer has already spread to my skin, until I'm an unusual, extreme case, to do anything. Suzy, my flatmate, noticed my inverted nipple a couple of weeks ago and said I should get it checked out, but I brushed off her concern. If only I hadn't. Ah well, I'm here now.

Back at the parental home, I sit in the garden. It's April and the great, coal and blue tits are flying to and from the feeders. *I don't want to die*, I think, watching them carrying food to their chicks. *It's spring. I don't want to die.* The plants and flowers seem so bright and fresh and new.

We arrive for the first day of chemotherapy. Mum is with me. I elect to try the cold cap. This is a cap of freezing nitrogen which I put on and it freezes the hair follicles. It has some success in 40 per cent of cases. I have beautiful long, dark brown curly hair and I don't want to lose it. I'm going to do everything within my power to keep my hair and my only option is this cold cap.

Sitting in the big blue chemo chair, the huge machine is wheeled over to me by a nurse. She brings a collection of caps, we find the one that fits me the closest and she attaches it to the tube of the machine. I put it on, and the pain is excruciating. I've taken a couple of ibuprofen already but it is So Cold that it makes my head ache a lot. I start crying. To my great relief, after half an hour my head goes numb.

"I'm sorry, we're going to have to try another vein," the nurse says. She's tried forcing a cannula into my arm, but chemotherapy makes your veins shrink away from the skin. After a couple more painful attempts she finds a vein and the drip starts to enter my body. It too feels cold.

I'm reading Kate Atkinson's *Life After Life*, about a Halifax pilot in the Second World War. I love her writing and the period – the novel starts in 1910 – and I'm able to concentrate on it now at last my head is numb. The first three chemotherapy sessions will be a drug called FEC (fluorouracil, epirubicin, cyclophosphamide). As well as causing the hair to fall out, this induces nausea and constipation. FEC is bright red and I'm surprised when I produce a fluorescent red wee in the hospital loo.

My mood is up, so I chat to nurses and the other patients. I notice some people are wheeling their chemo drips outside every so often. We're all arranged round the edges of a room. It transpires these people are wheeling their drips outside so they can smoke whilst undergoing chemotherapy!

My nineteen-year-old cat Romario – known as Furry – is in the last stages of kidney disease. He is dehydrated so Mum takes him to have water injected under his skin. I'm at my flat with my brother who's home from Abroad for the summer. Mum calls.

"Darling," Mum says. "I'm going to take Furry to the vet. I think it's time. Will you come with me?" Her voice is shaking, she sounds distraught.

"I can't," I say. I don't want to put myself through this. Selfish I know but I just can't.

"I'll go," my brother says, pulling on his coat. I hear the tap, tap of his cowboy boots receding and pour myself a glass of wine and then another with my lunch.

Two hours later the key turns in the door. It's my brother. He comes to sit with me in front of the television. He looks extremely upset.

"That was very sad," he says. "Poor Furry. I'm going to join you in a glass of wine."

He takes a glass down from the cupboard.

"What happened?" I ask, feeling bad I wasn't there.

"Mum held him," my brother says. There's a pause whilst he takes a sip of his wine. "Then the vet gave him an injection and he just went to sleep."

So that's it, I think. Dead, just like that, after nineteen years. He was a kitten of the 1994 World Cup, and he was black and white, like a football, so we named him Romario, after the Brazilian top goal scorer although we always called him Furry, and now he's gone.

By the next chemotherapy session, two weeks later, my mood has crashed. I feel so ill due to this horrible treatment – it's so real now. The panther makes me weak.

"Can you move my daughter into a bed, please?" Mum asks. "She's not well." Mum is miserable. I overhear her saying to a friend on the phone one day that Furry's death is worse than that of either of her parents.

They put me into one of the two beds in the room – for the weakest, most ill patients – and that's more comfortable. I can't talk to anyone. The panther lies on the bed next to me, resting his head on my shoulder. I'm reading a historical novel by Philippa Gregory, *The Queen's Fool*, about a converso in the court of Mary I who is in love with Robert Dudley and has second sight. I've stopped trying to read anything more difficult or anything about modern young women with lives so different from mine. Young women in peril, facing execution and war in the sixteenth century: that's the reading material I lap up in this period. My best friend Hannah sends me three of Philippa Gregory's Tudor Court novels for my birthday on the fifteenth of May and I work my way through them during chemotherapy.

The old people – apart from me everyone is old – laugh and joke with each other. Lying in my bed, cold cap holding my head in a vice, I don't want anyone to talk to me.

"They've had their lives," Mum says, looking devastated. This all has a terrible effect on her. She's aged twenty years in a mere few weeks: new lines etched on her tanned, beautiful face. I love Mum so much.

Chemotherapy on the National Health Service in West Herts, England, is an all-day process. We arrive after the morning rush hour – it's a forty-minute drive from Skybreak House and then we have to sit around for ages whilst they prepare my infusion. They don't start mixing your drugs until you've turned up, as they don't want to waste any drugs on patients who miss their appointments. The cold cap goes on thirty minutes before the infusion starts and stays on for an hour and a half after it ends. So, we're there all day.

The chap in the bed next to me is built like the proverbial brick shithouse and covered in tattoos. His wife, sitting at the foot of his bed, has long, platinum-blonde hair, is wearing dungarees and a pink t-shirt, and is also powerfully built with tattoos. They look frightening.

"She's such a darling," he says to a nurse, in a Watford accent. "She's deaf, but she's the cleverest little thing, my dog adores her. He was devastated when my last cat died, so little Rosie has cheered him up and …"

"Excuse me," I say. "Have you got a kitten?"

"A white one," he says, the expression on his face so soft it's amazing. "She's deaf. We got her from the rescue centre. She's such a sweet little thing." He breaks into a big smile.

He appears to be the most terrifying man, but I've never heard anyone be so in love with animals. One thing about NHS chemotherapy – you meet a real cross section of society. Despite the cold cap and the painful cannula insertion, I grow to enjoy my chemo days. The hospital is set in beautiful grounds – there's a garden behind the chemo wing in which we're not allowed, due to the threat of falling masonry from the ancient building, but it's beautiful and calming. I lie in my bed and read my Philippa Gregory books and am transported to Tudor England. Chemo is nowhere near as bad as I thought it would be.

My hair starts to fall out. At first, I'm able to move the remaining hair around to cover the bald patches. It falls out in clumps. As it works its way down it tangles up with hair that's still attached to form dreadlocks. Mum's bridge partner, who used to run a beauty salon, comes to help me and combs it through, removing a lot of hair but managing to detangle it.

I'm in Stratford-upon-Avon with Mum. We've driven to a birds of prey centre and we're driving back when there's a crunch and a deafening thud. Mum stops. A girl comes running towards us with a pack of borzois – four of them.

"My dog my dog," she screams, her face contorted with distress and horror.

By the side of the road, there's another borzoi, lying down. She can't get up.

"I didn't see her," Mum says, her voice shaking. "She was so fast I didn't see her. I love dogs. I can't believe …"

I look into the huge soft eyes of the dog in pain, at her long, elegant face. The girl and her father bundle her into their van.

The girl calls later to tell Mum that the dog's back is broken, and she has had her put down.

"Why did that have to happen?" Mum says through tears, as we sit on a bench outside the Swan Theatre, watching the white swans drifting on the lake: the peacefulness of this scene contrasting with the memory of the screech of brakes and the mangled dog.

Everything is against us.

Amid all the trauma, a good thing happens. Seb, the love of my life, who's been refusing to meet me since I got the cancer diagnosis in April as he's trying to be celibate, emails and says, "OK then, what harm can it do?" We agree to meet once I'm back from Stratford in September.

"You can't go around looking like that," my boss says, looking at me. I have strands of hair fixed with clips over the various bald patches. "I think it's time to get rid of your hair," she says.

"OK," I say.

We arrive at our local hairdresser, The Cutting Room. It's after hours and we have the place to ourselves. I'm crying – I'm dreading this. But then the hairdresser – a girl about my age – shaves my hair off and it's lying on The Cutting Room floor, and I look at it and I feel this enormous sense of freedom. My hair is gone, and I see now that it's just another thing I don't need. *I can wear my wig*, I think. My hair is gone, and I don't have to worry about it anymore, I don't have to comb it over bald patches. That's it. And this is such a profound realisation: I don't need it. I don't need anything. The less I'm carrying with me on my journey the better, as I fight to stay alive.

"I'm not going to charge you," the hairdresser says. *She must feel so sorry for me*, I think.

"Please let me give you something," Mum says.

"Just give me ten pounds," the girl says.

My wig is similar to my real hair but straight rather than curly: NHS hospitals have a service where each breast cancer patient is fitted for a wig. My one is brown, the same colour as my real hair. I have to wear a wig liner underneath it. But this is OK.

The Abraxane, the second sort of chemotherapy that I have because I can't have Taxol –you need to take steroids with Taxol and I can't due to the risk of psychosis with my mental disorder – seems to be working. When I see the oncologist, he feels the lump and it appears smaller to him. This is good as the FEC didn't seem to shrink the tumour at all, and we need it to be far, far, far smaller before surgery can take place.

Chapter 2

Seb comes to meet me at the pub near my flat. I haven't seen him for four years, not since 2009. He's lost weight – he's so thin now – and his hair is short: he had to shave it in the Buddhist monastery that he's been out of for a mere six months. It's amazing to see him after four years apart. Gazing into his remarkable, unusual turquoise eyes, I feel as in love with him as ever.

"My 'mum's cat is about to have kittens," Seb says, as we sip our drinks. I'm drinking Rioja and he's drinking Coke – he's still following the Buddhist precept forbidding him alcohol.

"Can I have one?" I ask.

He smiles at me. "Of course, I'll save the best one for you."

"Is it difficult, seeing me?"

"No, it's been lovely," he says, his voice mellifluous as ever. Seb used to be an actor and he has the most gorgeous voice. I go in for a kiss to say goodbye, but he won't kiss me as he's still trying to be celibate. I feel ecstatic: I know I'm going to see him again and I'm going to have one of his 'mum's kittens, so that will be a bond between us that will keep him coming back to me.

I have nine cycles of Abraxane in the end. After they've finished the first three, my oncologist decides to give me another six, as it seems to be shrinking the tumour. The Abraxane causes pain in my bones but I'm relieved to be delaying surgery: I've become used to chemotherapy and have started to dread the thought of surgery.

Seb meets me at Waterloo station, under the clock tower. We're catching the train to his 'mum's house for me to meet the kittens. Over the years I've imagined meeting his mum often, not in these circumstances: aged thirty-four, with breast cancer, not in a relationship with Seb, who is still refusing to kiss me as he's still trying to stay celibate.

I'm nervous about meeting Seb's Mum, and I put on a full face of make-up: blusher, lip gloss, eyeliner, even mascara. I'm wearing a short, long-sleeved black dress and tights and boots and it's hotter than I thought, so I'm sweating. I start crying.

"Why are you crying?" Seb asks, looking concerned, putting his hand on my arm.

"Well, you've told me so much about your mum," I say. "I'm a bit nervous and …"

"Don't worry," Seb says. "She likes most people."

There are six kittens: two black ones, a tortoiseshell one and three orange ones.

"I've picked this one for you," Seb says, putting the biggest orange one in my lap.

"What's he going to look like when he grows up?" I ask.

"He'll have a fluffy tail and long hair and a mane," Seb says. "Like his mum and uncle." The kitten's mum and uncle are named Kitty Hawk and Wellington, after the planes, and are pure-bred Ragdolls: cream with grey faces and tails, blue eyes, thick manes and long fur. They are so, so, so soft: it's stroking clouds.

As we play with the kittens, I gaze at Seb. Seb's Mum is beautiful: blonde and slim and glamorous. I wonder if she notices me staring at her son. I wonder what she thinks of me. *I love Seb*, I think.

We drive in torrential rain to pick the kitten up. Seb and his mum aren't there, just his stepdad. He gives us our kitten and we put him in the carrier and set off for home. The motorway traffic is terrible, and he cries all the way home. I put my hand into the top of the carrier to stroke him, but it doesn't stop his piteous howling.

"Don't open the top of that thing," Mum says from the front seat. "We don't want him to escape. Shhh Precious Angel Fluffball, it's OK – we're taking you home."

"Sorry," I say, closing the lid of the carrier.

As soon as we arrive home and put the box on the floor and open the door, the kitten strides out and starts exploring his bedroom as if he owns the place. Whether it's the effect of the Feliway pheromone diffuser or just his personality, he's not timid at all. He's on a mission – stomping about, inquisitive, this little orange ball of fluff. So here he is. My life-saving kitten.

The humans in his family are pilots so their animals are all named after planes and pilots: his aunts' are Fatby and Chinook. The dogs are Bomber, Buster and Doodle. Because he's orange – the colour of fire – and because it's the most beautiful plane, I decide to call the kitten Spitfire, to keep him in touch with his roots.

I'm in a meeting with my breast surgeon after my nine cycles of chemotherapy.

"I'm just going to call the plastic surgeon who will perform the operation with me," she says, picking up her mobile phone. I hear it ringing.

"Oh, hello," she says. "Do you remember me telling you about that extreme case – the girl with the tumour in her skin and … yes, you do. Well, I'm with her now and we'd like to arrange a time to meet and …"

Extreme case, I think. *I am an extreme case.* On one level I've known this since the start of the whole business but it's strange to hear it confirmed: even by my surgeon, who must see so many patients. We've decided I'm going to go private for the operation, because it means I can have the plastic surgeon as well as my breast surgeon doing the operation together, and because I'll be in hospital for about a week I think I'll need the privacy of my own room: I don't want to be stuck on a ward with lots of old people. From this point onwards, my treatment is a mixture of NHS and private healthcare.

Mum, Dad and I are in a consultation with my breast surgeon and the plastic surgeon, who will perform the operation. A plastic surgery nurse in a white coat hovers in the background behind a trolley of bandages, plasters, syringes and so on. The two doctors are on one side of the desk and my parents and I are on the other side. He's a round, cheerful man with a big smile. I feel at ease with him straight away.

"So," he says, looking at me. "If you just go behind the curtain, please, and slip your top things off."

"OK," I say. Behind the curtain is a bed and I lie down on it.

The plastic surgeon and the nurse follow me behind the curtain.

"Tape measure, please," he says to the nurse, and she hands it to him. He squeezes my tummy. "Not a lot of spare flesh here," he says.

"Thank you," I say. *I've put on half a stone with the chemotherapy*, I think.

He examines my right breast and takes some measurements on my tummy and back.

"Alright," he says, smiling at me. "You can put your things back on and come back to the table."

Putting my top back on, I return to my seat next to Mum.

"You see, the thing is," he says. "If I remove all the cancerous skin, you're not going to have enough skin even to close the gap, let alone to make a new breast."

"Oh," I say.

"There is one thing we can try," he says. He turns to my breast surgeon, and they exchange a couple of sentences in a whisper.

"So," he says, looking at me. "There's something called a skin expander which will stretch the skin on your back. It will be inserted under the skin, and we'll blow it up by putting a hundred millilitres of saline in it every week, over six weeks, and then it will be big enough to replace the skin we'll remove from your front. In the operation, I'll just move it to your front and it will become a new breast."

I look at Mum and Dad. Our jaws drop.

"That sounds medieval," I say. "I don't want to grow a hump on my back." It sounds awful.

"It was invented to treat pilots who had been shot down and suffered terrible burns in the First World War," he says. "They used to grow the humps on their faces and ..."

"OK," I say. "I'll do it."

"Why do I have to have such a horrible treatment?" I ask Mum, once we're in the car.

"I don't know, darling," Mum says.

"It's amazing there's something they can do," Dad says.

I go into hospital to have the expander inserted. When I come round from the anaesthetic I'm in pain and there's a small hump behind my right shoulder. Each week, I return to the hospital to have more saline pumped into it. After each treatment I feel the skin stretching so I am in constant pain throughout the six weeks. We call my hump Engelbert, after Engelbert Humperdink. My best friend Mary suggests the name. I grow quite attached to him – he's the shape of half a ball under my skin and after each saline injection the skin hurts as he expands. But Engelbert comes everywhere with me, and I grow to regard him with fondness.

I attend Christmas dinner at my aunt's house wearing a black Ted Baker dress accessorised with red lipstick, turquoise eyeliner and a hump on my back. The operation is scheduled for the eighth of January 2014 – the plastic surgeon decides Engelbert is now big enough. It's going to be a transverse rectus abdominis mycocutaneous flap operation (TRAM flap) where my right breast will be sliced off and a new one constructed from my hump and a portion of my back muscle underneath the implant.

Chapter 3

2014

"I need a wee," I say. I'm wobbly. I've come round from an eight-hour operation and I must do a wee. Stumbling into the bathroom, I collapse on the floor with a heavy thud, tangled in the tubes of my three drain bottles. A nurse picks me up, helps me onto the loo. Out of the corner of my eye I can see Mum looking worried. On the loo, at last, I do a long elephant wee. Two nurses help me back into bed. I have a drain coming out of the wound on my back and two at the side of my chest. These are to catch the blood and fluid that is seeping from my wounds. There are stitches all the way around my right breast where it has been removed and replaced with the skin from Engelbert.

I'm in hospital for eight days this first time. Every evening Dad comes to sit with me, and we watch Hitchcock films. The combination of morphine and Hitchcock is a good one. I have a drip at the beginning and when I click a button more morphine is delivered into my bloodstream. On the first night I'm talking to Mary on the phone when the walls start to move: a hallucinatory effect of the drug.

On Friday night, both my parentals come to the hospital for dinner, and we watch *North by Northwest*.

"I'm going to remove two of your drains now," the nurse says. "Breathe in."

Oh, it hurts, it hurts so much – especially the one which is curled around my wound. Ouch. On the plus side, I can go home, after eight days, although I still have one drain – the one coming out of the huge wound in my back. They give me codeine to take home, not morphine which is such a shame. I love morphine. My life goal is to be at an opium den down at the docks with Sherlock Holmes. The Lascar lets us in, and he waits behind the curtain. I lie on my back on a mat next to Sherlock, dribbling, paralysed by the drug. When Seb was a posh teenage boy, he broke into Kew Gardens with his chums and they removed opium poppies and smoked the drug. *Darling Seb, come back to me for ever*, I pray.

At home, I'm in so much pain. The codeine isn't enough to stop this so my doctors prescribe a stronger drug, tramadol. I shuffle around in my dressing gown with the drain bottle tucked into my pocket. Spitfire chases the long, twisting tube of the drain as it moves and, being a kitten, attempts to catch it.

Chapter 4

I suffer from bipolar disorder, otherwise known as manic depression. Or, to put it another way: I am bipolar or I am a manic depressive. I've had this illness in some form since I was nineteen years old, so perhaps I should've started this memoir with when I first became mentally ill. Far more than the cancer ever could, the bipolar forms an integral part of my personality. I've been a manic depressive for my whole adult life: the illness affects me every day in countless ways. It's a crucial part of my identity. I've made friends through bipolar support groups. I'm in films, television and radio programmes about my bipolar disorder and how it affects me. It forms the main subject of most of my writing: in fact the hypomania – the phase of my illness when I'm not depressed – is the engine of my writing.

This is how I experience the illness: My mood is up – hypomanic – for around four and a half to six months, although my most recent high lasted eight months. During this period, I wake at 3 a.m. or 5 a.m. on a late day, have boundless energy and am on the phone and the internet non-stop. I write pages and pages. My strength and stamina in Pilates and barre classes are impressive and I put my weights up in classes and personal training. Wearing bright colours, I'm always taking my clothes off. I'm an exhibitionist and uninhibited, cracking constant jokes. I make many plans with friends and spend so much money buying dresses, jewellery and books. I feel happy and content with my life and my head is full of plans and ideas. My parents worry so much about my spending.

Other people think I'm "on good form" but I'm irritable with my parents as they can't keep up with the speed of my thoughts. I fall asleep late and wake up with the dawn, eager to crack on with the day. I talk to everyone, striking up conversations with strangers and chatting to shopkeepers as I'm always in shops, spending money. This mood state seems divinely ordained. I feel my mood will stay up forever, that I'm cured of my depression.

Another place where I could have started this memoir is when I end up in a police station aged twenty-four, saying I've been raped. I've been out on a five-day bender, it's the Bank Holiday at the end of May 2003 and I've been out clubbing four nights running, not even going home in between. I don't know how I've ended up here – that's mania for you, it wipes the memory. Thankfully, in many cases. But this is where my cyclothymia – the embryonic form of bipolar – becomes bipolar 1 – the most severe kind. After the police station, I'm in the mental hospital for six weeks and for the first four I'm in the tight grip of mania – I don't receive the anti-manic drugs until my mood is already sky-high, and by then it's too late to bring it down. You can't be diagnosed bipolar 1 unless you've been hospitalised with mania, and now I have.

After the drugs bring my mood down at long last, I'm in hospital for another couple of weeks as Mum's a schoolteacher and she won't let them send me home until she's around to look after me during her summer holiday. And after I receive the bipolar 1 diagnosis, my whole life is changed forever. I attend the STEADY programme (Support and Training for Elation and Depression in Youth), run by what was then the Manic Depression Fellowship" and later became Bipolar UK. And I make friends there, including Corey who's still a good friend, and then join the MDF's internet message board, where

I make yet more new friends, including my best friend Mary and good chum Becky. And because the STEADY programme is funded by Comic Relief, I do some media work for them: the first piece in a series that continues to this day.

And then, one day I wake up and my mood has changed. I'm depressed: the panther is here. It's as sudden as a switch flicking. I don't want to get out of bed. Mum hauls me up, but when I'm exercising I'm so weak and I can't put my weights up. I don't want to talk to anyone. I keep my head down. I can't look anyone in the eye. I don't bother with make-up and dress in black. The panther is always with me. He tells me I'm fat and useless, that I can't write. I don't enter shops or try on clothes. My thoughts are slow, and I don't understand things. Every night I lie in bed, hoping I won't wake up the next morning. I pray for death. When I was younger, I made several suicide attempts which increased in severity. I didn't stop until my cancer diagnosis.

My most recent depression lasted for six months and I'm scared that the one I'm in now will drag on that long as well. A few years ago, I changed mood stabilisers from carbamazepine to lurasidone, which is licensed for bipolar in the USA: here it's just licensed for schizophrenia. I also changed antidepressants from duloxetine back to venlafaxine, which is a stronger SNRI (selective serotonin and norepinephrine reuptake inhibitor). I'm not allowed SSRI (selective serotonin reuptake inhibitor) antidepressants such as Prozac and citalopram as there's a danger they can operate what's called "the manic switch" – best explained as adding a positive to a positive, making one's mood go extra high into full-blown mania, which is what I experienced in the mental hospital aged twenty-four and never want to suffer again. Mania destroys lives and can kill: I have had friends who have jumped off bridges and cliffs and under trains to their deaths.

This time my mood is not as low as it has been in the past, and my coping strategies are better now – I've been dealing with this illness for twenty years and have been seeing my wonderful psychiatrist Dr Joshua Stein privately for that whole time, so of course I've learnt some coping strategies along the way.

Coping Strategies for When I'm Depressed

- Set an alarm and, whether I feel like it or not, wake up, have breakfast and attend a Pilates or barre class on Zoom. It's vital to haul myself up and out in the morning or I know I will feel even worse. Dr Stein first told me this when I was twenty-two. Waking at the same time every day helps regulate my behaviour.
- Write the blog every day. It's cathartic and it gives me a sense of achievement. I have an Instagram account for my tarot business now: @TaurusSunAndMercuryTarot. Please follow it if you are so inclined.
- Bathe. At least once a week, even if I don't feel like it, which I don't.
- Stay in contact with friends. When the panther is here, he likes to keep me to himself, but it improves my mood to see people, although it's the last thing I want to do and I have to push myself hard to achieve this.
- Knit. This is calming and gives me something to focus on.
- Read: my concentration is better when my mood is low and so I can focus on a book all day and escape from my horrible reality.
- Exercise: endorphins give my mood a temporary boost.
- Visit London Zoo. I worked there in my gap year, and it always cheers me up to see the sloths, otters and tamanduas, lions, tigers and penguins, hyacinth macaws, toucans and hummingbirds. All animals are my favourites.

- Cuddle my cat, Spitfire.
- If my mood is rock bottom: stay at my parental home so Mum can feed me, drag me out of bed for Pilates and barre and look after me. Also, it helps to know the parentals are there even if they are in another room and that Spitfire is there too, my cuddle monster.
- Watch or read a Golden Age of Crime murder mystery: *Poirot, Miss Marple, Inspector Morse, Foyles War* or *Midsomer Murders*: a traditional English murder where I know all the loose ends will be tied up and order will be restored.

My mood is low and I don't have much energy so I'm sitting up in bed typing this. I know I'll feel better once I've finished the two thousand words I've set myself for today. It is a struggle: writing when the panther is here. He lies next to me and whispers "You can't write, nobody will want to read it, it's boring." But I must just ignore him and keep going.

Coping Strategies for When My Mood Is Up

- Don't make too many plans.
- Go to bed at a sensible time. Make sure to listen to a body scan meditation in bed to relax myself. Read if sleep eludes me.
- Turn phone off and make sure it's not in my bedroom at night.
- Keep out of clothes shops.
- Keep away from dangerous situations.
- Be careful when crossing roads: the cars won't bend round me, even if I think they will.
- Make sure to eat three meals a day.
- Don't spend too much time on the phone.
- Avoid too much caffeine.

- Avoid arguing with strangers on the internet. Keep off Facebook and social media as much as possible.

Because the panther is here at the moment, it's impossible to remember how it feels not to be depressed, when I know my thoughts would be faster and I would have more confidence and far more energy, but at the moment, this depression seems permanent: *I deserve to be suicidal, my life has no meaning or purpose, I deserve to feel like this and I will always feel like this*. Mum says that I'm two different people: a high one and a low one. It's impossible for her ever to become acclimatised to this which is tough on all of us: all our lives are controlled by my mental disorder and have been for more than twenty years now.

The form of the illness I have, "rapid cycling" – two or more mood cycles per year – means I'm always ill. In classic bipolar, someone will have a big high, then a big low, followed by a period of normal mood. I don't have that. I'm always either depressed, hypomanic or manic. There is never a day when I'm not suffering from the effects of hypomania, mania or depression. There is never a day when I don't think about my mental disorder.

A psychologist, Jan Scott, once said to me that bipolar disorder is the mental illness where there's the greatest gap between ability and achievement. I lost my first job when I suffered my first full-blown manic episode when I was twenty-four, and then, after six weeks in the mental hospital I landed another entry-level position. Starting off full-time, I cut down to part-time and over the next thirteen years I worked two, three then two and finally one day per week. In 2016, I started my dream job in a book shop but lasted just three days there before the shop closed. Now, I am a successful tarot reader with a published novel and training to be an astrologer.

Perhaps without bipolar I would have made more of my writing. Over the years I've had long periods of depression when I couldn't write. After my agent sent out my first novel and it was rejected by all the publishers we tried, I couldn't write again for about four years. It took the NaNoWriMo challenge to start me writing again, and then starting my first blog to force me into the habit of writing every day. I also have long periods of hypomania where I start projects and abandon them when my mood crashes, or write pages and pages of rubbish. I find it impossible to work consistently at my writing because a mood disorder is the worst enemy of consistency. Every time my mood rockets I purchase art supplies and draw and paint non-stop, then give them all away when my mood crashes. Mania is horrifying and ruinous: I spend all my savings when manic, then crash and am broke again.

It is probable that without bipolar, I would have settled down with a partner. Boyfriends have found my mood swings impossible to cope with. I find looking after myself more than I can deal with much of the time, never mind considering someone else. I know Seb was unable to deal with my mental disorder. I have often become involved with unsuitable people: a few years ago, when I was thirty-seven, I dated a twenty-three-year-old musician. More on him later. There have been addicts, alcoholics and chaps who just weren't that into me. I've also dated other manic depressives – bad mistake.

On the other hand, my mental disorder has brought some good things into my life.

Good Things Bipolar Has Brought Me

- My wonderful psychiatrist Dr Joshua Stein who I've been seeing privately since I was twenty-two years old.
- Various hypomanic obsessions which have led to interests in Formula One, Leonard Cohen, the First World War, Golden

Age detective fiction, serial killers, Nazis, abandoned shipwrecks and countless other areas of study.

- Daily meditation practice.
- Weightlifting, Schwinn cycling and barre to lift my mood, to work off hypomanic energy, to achieve something by lifting heavier and heavier weights.
- The ability to wring every last bit of enjoyment out of my life.
- The coping strategies I've employed to help me manage my bipolar symptoms have allowed me to deal with the brutal cancer treatments and their side effects.
- Much of my writing has been done during hypomanic periods and the confidence to read it out loud at events is the confidence of hypomania.
- I published my first novel which was a real dream come true. I also narrated my own audiobook.

It's possible, of course, that my personality and my thirst to write would have stopped me from having a career anyway. But I bet the fact I've never taken work with any seriousness, and have always taken relationships with the utmost seriousness, is down to my mental disorder. I can't go back and live my twenties and thirties again, but what I can do, starting now, is to write two thousand words a day, rewrite, edit and just make sure I finish the damn thing. Life begins at forty after all.

It's a sunny, mid-September day in 2019 as I edit this sixth draft, lying on cushions in the garden. I don't miss work, that's for sure as I Google Rafael Nadal's diet and exercise regime. I'm a Rafaholic and following tennis is one of the great joys of my life, so much so that I purchase Amazon Prime in order to watch the US Open in August. I watch every single match. Darling Rafa wins the title in a five-set thriller defeating the up and coming twenty-three-year-old Russian

Daniil Medvedev 6–4 in the fifth. I'm now a founder member of a Rafaholics' WhatsApp group where we discuss our Greatest of All Time, now just one Grand Slam title behind the great Roger Federer's twenty. We're in a wonderful era of men's tennis as the big three – Rafa, Roger and Novak spur each other on to ever greater record-breaking feats.

Film Chap loves tennis too and I'm happy that he visits me at the flat so we can watch Sunday's final together, although he has to leave at midnight to sleep in preparation for the office on Monday. Long may the reign of the big three continue: we're privileged to be living in their era and they seem to be, if anything, improving with age: adding new shots to their repertoires with alarming regularity. I don't think a Grand Slam has been won by a man under thirty this century, such is the hold the big three have on the game. Long may they continue to awe and inspire us.

Chapter 5

2014

"Arms above your head, that's right," the radiologist's voice penetrates the sound system into the room. I'm lying on a board on my back with a foam block behind me. My arms are lifted. My wrists are held in clamps. My top half is naked. "Hold still," she says. The machine above me whirrs round and fires a bolt at me, although I feel nothing. This is radiotherapy and, because I have cancer in my skin, I must have three times the normal dose.

"Ok, we're going to go again," the radiologist says. Again, a bolt is fired. I see nothing except the huge machine above me spinning round to change position.

"Good girl," she says. "Now we're going to strap on the bolus." This is a heavy gel sheet which is strapped on to my chest with strips of sticky tape which allows the rays not only to be diffused over a wider area but also to penetrate deeper into the skin. As I lie on the board, blanket over my feet: it's cold in here, the bolus presses down on me.

Again, the machine whirrs and changes position. It fires radiation at me.

"Ok, all done," the radiologist says.

Another radiologist enters the room – the one who strapped me into the machine at the session's start. Removing the tape from my side, chest and shoulders, she takes the bolus off me.

"All done," she says, smiling. She wears a blue uniform and has long brown hair streaked with caramel highlights and a mellifluous voice. "See you tomorrow."

"Thank you. See you tomorrow," I say, putting my secret support top back on, leaving the room. Mum is waiting for me in the waiting room, doing *The Times* crossword.

"How was it, darling?" she asks, eyes wide with concern.

"Yeah, fine," I say.

Mum drives me home. The hospital is just a ten-minute drive away which is good as radiotherapy will be every day, except Saturday and Sunday, for five weeks. We decided to go private for radiotherapy as NHS radiotherapy takes place at the hospital where I had chemo, a forty-minute drive each way from home. This would be too exhausting every day for five weeks. Another bonus of the private hospital is I can choose when during the day to have my radiotherapy and have opted for after the gym in the morning, around eleven o'clock.

The operation was at the start of January, but my skin needed to heal up so now we're in mid-February 2014.

I sleep after lunch. I'm very tired. When I wake up, I watch *Poirot* with Dad and Spitfire. My Precious Angel Fluffball sits on his pink chair near the television and rests, eyes closed, his tail wrapped around his paws.

Every morning, I attend the gym and lift weights. Then Mum or Dad takes me to radiotherapy. The session takes about twenty minutes but there's always traffic, or a queue of people at the hospital, so the whole business can take an hour or even an hour and a half.

After two weeks, my skin is red and sore and begins to peel off. At the start it looks sunburnt and its condition continues to deteriorate. Now, during radiotherapy, I feel my damaged skin sizzling. By the end of the five weeks, I have deep burns all over my chest and under my arm: my skin has broken down. Mum takes me to the hospital where the breast care nurse shows her how to dress my third degree burns and gives us pads to keep my top away from them. I have to use the pink Micropore tape from the plastic surgery unit. Since chemotherapy I've become allergic to most of the dressings they try to use on me. The pink Micropore tape is fine but the white one uses a different glue which gives me a terrible rash. Most of the dressings have plastic parts to which I'm allergic, so Mum has to pack my wounds with gauze and stick this onto my skin with the pink Micropore tape.

During this time, I'm allowed to sit in the bath, as long as I keep my dressings dry. Mum washes my hair over the bath, and I collapse with dizziness. The radiotherapy exhausts me.

In some ways, this isn't a bad time. I know what I'm doing every day: gym then radiotherapy. A friend lends Mum the first Rebus book, and we devour all of them, escaping into the criminal underbelly of Ian Rankin's Edinburgh. It's spring by the time radiotherapy finishes and we sit on the swinging chair in the garden, reading Rebus.

That spring and summer, I have to wear a scarf and hat as I mustn't expose my irradiated skin to the sun.

In April, just after the end of radiotherapy, I attend a weekend for Young Women with Breast Cancer, run by Breast Cancer Care. The panther is with me, and I find it devastating hearing all the ways in which breast cancer has impacted all these women's lives. There's a veterinary nurse who can't work anymore: if an animal bites or scratches her, she could develop lymphoedema. Each girl has had their life ripped apart by this illness. There's a session where we do a body scan and one about relationships. Most of the women are older than me and have husbands and children, but there are a few other single ones. One of the girls recounts telling a man on a date that she's wearing a wig. An idea starts to form in my head. The last session is about nutrition, and I skip it to leave early. I've found the whole weekend too depressing.

My best friend Mary starts a blog about running.

"Why don't I write a blog about dating after breast cancer surgery," I say to my brother who is at the flat with me visiting from Abroad. "It will mean I have to go on dates and write about them. It will be work. You know, dating wearing a wig and false eyelashes and wearing clothes that cover my scars and …"

"Good idea," my brother says, smiling, stroking his beard. "Where are you going to find the men?"

"Well, there's this new phone app called Tinder which a couple of my male friends are raving about," I say. "You don't need to fill in a form about how you want to educate your children, nothing about religious observance" (we're Jewish and the only internet dating I've done before is the Jewish website J Date). "You just make a profile with a picture. You don't have to tell people anything about yourself or …"

"Sounds perfect," my brother says smiling his huge grin at me. I love to impress him which becomes harder and harder as he becomes more and more successful and critical.

I decide to call the blog *Scars, Tears and Training Bras*. It's anonymous. I call myself Tanya in it: the name of the protagonist in my first novel, *In Bloom.*

I build up a long list of prospects on Tinder. The average age of the app's users is twenty-seven so most of my boys are far younger than me. It's addictive. I love swiping left and right on the profiles. It's a sweetshop of boys: shallow and fun and a world away from cancer treatment. I wonder how I'm going to feel, dressing up, pulling on my wig, pretending to be normal.

I'm in the bar of the Churchill Hotel in town, near Marble Arch, wearing a new dress that comes up to my neck, covering the scars on my chest. It's from Wallis and emblazoned with flowers in bright colours: orange, cobalt, lime green. It's tight and knee-length. I'm waiting for my first date: he's a trainee doctor. Sitting outside, next to the statue of Churchill on a bench, I observe him approach: he has a mop of blond hair.

I needn't have worried, conversation flows. He flies small planes for fun and he tells me about this and about his medical training. He's polite, charming and fascinating: I have a wonderful time. *This is great*, I think: *I'm out, dressed up and enjoying myself, drinking champagne cocktails with a twenty-six-year-old man*. Anyway, when I walk back to Baker Street I'm cheerful.

When I've written a mere couple of blogs, Mumsnet ask me to write a guest post for their website. At my best friend's urging, I've linked the blog up to the Mumsnet Bloggers' Network. I write my post and it appears on the website to acclaim but also criticism: "Why am I dating such young men?" the Mumsnetters demand.

I achieve many first dates and enjoy them. My mood is up at this time, so I'm charming and talkative and relish meeting the chaps and asking them where they grew up and so on: there's a lot of foreign bankers. I have a set routine for most of the dates. For safety reasons I ask them to meet me at my local pub and after a drink I take them round the park where there are animals: coatis, lemurs, maras, kookaburras, donkeys and Lady Amherst's pheasants. They all tell me it's the best date they've ever been on.

Various dates express a desire to see me again, but when it comes down to it, I don't hear from them. At the start I'm going on several dates a week: it's summer and I can walk to the pub in half an hour from my flat, knock back a drink or two, walk around the park and be home before dark.

Despite the lack of second dates, I find myself loving both the dating and the resultant blogging. I'm writing the blog every day, so it becomes a record of this time, containing meetings with my doctors and my psychiatrist Dr Stein, as well as narratives of the dates and vignettes of my life with my parents, brother and Spitfire.

In August I attend a writing holiday in Burgundy. It's at a beautiful farm with a swimming pool. During the day we work on our writing and in the evenings, we consume a marvellous three-course dinner and chat and sometimes read out our work.

I've been swimming and I'm lying in the bath in my private bathroom at the writing retreat. Looking down at my chest I see what appears to be a rash, but I just *know* it's not. I know the cancer has come back. I call my dad.

"Dad," I say. "I'm sorry to disturb you on your holiday, but I think the cancer has come back on my chest."

"Are you sure," Dad says. The line crackles – they're in France too.

"Yes, I'm sure," I say. "It looks the same as it did before, it's just around my scar and …"

"OK," Dad says, sounding worried. "I'll try to get in touch with your doctors but it's August they'll be away and …"

"I'm sorry to ruin your holiday," I say, looking down at what I know is cancer on my chest.

"It's OK," Dad says, sounding resigned. "You had to tell us. Thank you for letting me know. I'll get onto your oncologist's secretary straight away."

"Bye Dad," I say.

"Goodbye. Try not to worry," Dad says in his best ever calm, look-how-long-suffering-I-am voice. I stare at my chest.

The Kraken wakes, I write in the blog. The Kraken wakes and stirs under my skin reaching his long tentacles through my capillaries. The cancer is back. The break I've had for a mere few months after treatment is over and I will need more surgery. After my initial operation my breast surgeon said she'd removed as much of the tumour as possible but there hadn't been any spare skin to leave margins. There was always the possibility the cancer would come back in the skin and now here it is, ruining both my holiday and my parents'. Life is cruel.

Chapter 6

2015

"The results of the punch biopsies are back," my breast surgeon says. I'm sitting with Mum in my doctor's consulting room. "And I'm afraid they show the skin is cancerous."

"It looks just like it did before," Mum says, sounding shaken. "Thank you. We suspected as much."

"Once skin has had cancer in it, it will keep coming back," my breast surgeon says. "And I'm afraid I didn't take away enough skin the first time – there was just enough skin to cover the hole left by the amount of tissue we had to remove: leaving clear margins wasn't possible. It was always a possibility this would happen. I'm sorry, it's my fault."

No, it's my fault, I think. *It's my fault as usual.*

Looking down at the cancer spreading away from my scar, I see it swallowing up my whole body: an army of cancer cells advancing across the vast darkening plains of my skin.

"You're going to need another operation, I'm afraid," my breast surgeon says, swishing her mane of long, glossy dark hair. She's wearing a yellow shift dress and is glamorous as always. "If you book that with your plastic surgeon – he's not as busy as I am so …"

"Of course," Mum says. "Dad will get hold of his secretary," she says, turning to me.

Leaving the NHS Breast Care Clinic, we walk down the hill towards the car. Thinking about yet more surgery I look up at the sky.

"Look, Mum," I say, pointing above our heads to where there's a red kite circling: a flash of red tummy and a forked tail.

"What a beautiful person," Mum says gazing upwards. "Don't worry, darling, Dad and I will look after you." She puts her arm round me and we watch the raptor drift on the thermals. Everything is still and silent in this perfect moment.

I'm surfacing from a deep pool. Opening my mouth, I gulp for air. Opening my eyes, I see I'm in the Recovery room at the hospital. I'm in so much pain in my chest that I start crying big gulping sobs. I push away the oxygen mask that covers my nose and mouth.

"Morphine," I say. I know the nurses have it and I need some because it hurts so much.

"There, there," a nurse says, squirting a syringe of sickly-sweet Oramorph into my mouth. She passes me a plastic cup of water. "Drink this."

"I want my mum," I say, through gulping sobs.

"I'll call your mum and tell her you've come round from the anaesthetic and someone will take you back to your room soon," the nurse says. She is a large lady with a big smile and a reassuring voice. "You have to stay here for a bit though."

"I want my mum," I say, crying. "I want my mum."

In the bed across from me, there is an older woman. She is breathing through a tube and her eyes are closed. She is in a bad way. I want to get out of here, but I can't move – I'm helpless. I watch the woman opposite me breathing through her tube whilst the tears roll down my face.

"I can come and see you on Sunday," Seb says when he calls. It's mid-February.

"But I've got work on Monday," I say.

"That can't be helped," Seb says. "I can stay the night."

"See you then," I say, feeling excited as I put down the phone.

The last couple of times Seb has visited, we've kissed. He seems to have relaxed his position on celibacy.

I put on make-up and a dress whilst I wait for Seb at the flat. Applying my Nars Super Orgasm blusher, I look at my reflection. I look alright. I'm wearing a long, bright red wig tied up in a ponytail and my eyebrows and lashes have grown back. I ring my eyes with black glittery Nars pencil liner.

The buzzer goes. He's here. I slip on my high, black rubber Melissa shoes and open the door.

"Hello," he drawls, enveloping me in a hug. Resting my head on his chest, I breathe in his scent. He's six foot three, just the right amount taller than me. I feel delicate and protected in his arms. He's put on a bit of weight now he's eating three meals a day again – when he first left the monastery he was eating just once a day.

"Come in," I say, taking his hand, gazing into those turquoise eyes. I love him so much.

We watch a silly werewolf film – *The Wolfman* with Benicio del Toro, Anthony Hopkins and Emily Blunt – lying in the nest in front of the television, made from pushing both the sofa beds together to make one bed. We eat takeaway pizza and kiss. Then we retire to the bedroom. Modesty dictates that I shut the bedroom door behind us.

Waking up the next morning with Seb in my bed, I'm so happy.

"So," I say, sitting up in bed. "Now that we're together, we are together, aren't we?"

"Yes," Seb drawls.

"So, um, I'm going to stop the dating," I say, looking into the mirror so I can see his facial expression, gauge his reaction.

"Yes, I would prefer that," Seb says, in a definite tone of voice.

We dress and catch the bus to my office. Sitting next to Seb I'm so happy.

Outside the office, we're embracing when my colleague's mum walks past. She cleans at the office.

"Hello," she says, looking at Seb.

"Um, hi," I say. "This is Seb, he's…um…he's my boyfriend."

"Nice to meet you Seb," she says, smiling, and disappears down the stairs into the basement.

Seb starts laughing, his turquoise eyes crinkle at the corners and puts his arms round me. "You're so cute," he says. "Have a good day – I'll see you soon."

"I'm afraid it's not good news," my oncologist says. I'm sitting in his office with Mum. It's early in March.

"What is it?" Mum looks worried.

"I've got the biopsy results and the scan results here, and I'm afraid the cancer has spread," he says. "There are ductal carcinomas in your other breast and there appears to be cancer in your lungs."

"Are you sure?" I ask, shocked.

"Well, we can't be sure about the deposits in your lungs without doing a biopsy, but it looks cancerous," he says.

"Could you remove a section of lung?" Mum asks,

"No, I'm afraid that won't be possible as the cancer is diffuse over the surfaces of both lungs," he says.

"So, what do we do now?" Mum asks, holding my hand, looking at the oncologist. This sounds bad. I'm feeling shock, and also that a part of me always knew it could go like this.

"Well, now that there's secondary cancer we have to start on an aromatase inhibitor," he says, turning to look at me. "But first we have to give you a Zoladex injection to put you into the menopause. We can do that here."

"And do the studies show good results for this treatment?" Mum says, sounding worried.

"There's no literature dealing with what she's got," he says. "The literature only goes up to two years with what *she's* got and…"

"And I've had those two years already," I say. It's March 2015 now and I was diagnosed in April almost two years before.

"We have to try the Zoladex and the aromatase inhibitor," he says. "You've had so much chemotherapy already that you can't have any more. This is the only thing left to try."

"Is it weight neutral?" I ask. I'm terrified of gaining weight and have been known to refuse drugs that cause weight gain. I sense I don't have that option here.

He just laughs.

"If you lie down here," my Macmillan nurse says, gesturing towards the bed. "I can do the Zoladex injection now."

I go behind the curtain and climb onto the bed, lying on my back.

"Just lift your top up," she says. "It has to go into your tummy."

The needle comes towards me, it's huge – knitting needle size. It punctures my side and I flinch away from it. "No, it hurts too much," I say.

"OK," the breast care nurse says. "I'll put some numbing cream on but it will take half an hour to work and…"

"Can I call my boyfriend?" I ask.

"Of course," she says.

The Macmillan nurse takes Mum and me into a small private room. There is information about aromatase inhibitors that Mum starts to read. I dial Seb's number.

"Seb," I say.

"Yes?" he says. "What is it?"

"The cancer has spread, and I want to visit you," I say. "My cousin will bring me and…"

"Of course, my darling," he says, his voice shaking with emotion. "I finish term on the twenty-fifth so after that. I'll stay with you *'til the end*, if it comes to that."

"Thank you," I say. "I'll speak to my cousin and we'll come and see you on the twenty-eighth – he'll drive us."

I'm in the car with my cousin Patrick and his wife Julia, on our way to see Seb. I'm wearing a dress I know he likes, my short grey sleeveless one from Nolita, emblazoned with a huge, sequinned macaw, and worn with tights and boots because it's March and it's still cold. As we travel down to Worthing in the car, I'm excited. I can't wait to see my darling Seb.

He's waiting for us at the restaurant. He envelops me in a huge hug and I'm so happy to be with him. Seb and I sit on one side of the table next to each other and my cousin takes a photo of us.

After lunch we go for a walk to the pier. It's a grey day and it's raining and green waves lash against the shore and the sides of the pier.

"This is what the seaside's meant to be like – the proper English seaside," Patrick says, loudly, over the sound of the crashing waves. "Not like that rubbish beach in Barbados."

We all laugh.

We drive to Brighton and walk around. My cousin takes photos of Seb and me standing in front of some of the graffiti. We have an early dinner at the famous vegetarian restaurant Terre *à* Terre. It's a wonderful meal. Afterwards, they drop us back at Seb's flat in Worthing.

"I've got something for you," Seb says, handing me a little box. Opening it, I see it's a silver necklace with a small silver disc pendant engraved with a flower.

"Oh, darling, I love it," I say, putting the necklace on and smiling at my boyfriend.

I stay with Seb all week, phoning up to cancel my Monday and Tuesday office days. One sunny day, we walk to the beach. Worthing has a sandy beach, unlike the stony one in Brighton. We sit on the sand and the seagulls form a ring around us. We put our arms round each other and gaze out to sea. My happiness is complete. My cancer has spread and yet I've never felt so blessed. G-d has answered my prayers and brought Seb back to me.

Walking along the sea front, we come across a Turkish restaurant.

"Let's go here," I say.

"Sure," Seb says.

We sit outside. We order falafel, hummous, chips, tzatziki, a Greek salad and a couple of glasses of wine. We're both drinking quite a lot. Seb has abandoned his no-drinking Buddhist precept, as well as the one about no sexual activity.

"Don't eat all the tzatziki," Seb says. "I like to have some with my chips."

"OK, darling," I say, looking out to sea. "Isn't this wonderful, I'm so happy."

"Me too," Seb says. "This is a surprise for me – this isn't what I planned for this year, but I'm really happy too."

After lunch we go back to Seb's flat. It's a studio flat near the beach.

"I'm going to cover up the statue of the Buddha. The Buddha mustn't see us doing sexuals" Seb says. "And all my Buddhist texts." He puts a scarf over his Buddha statue which sits above the bed looking down on us, so he can't see what we're about to do, and another scarf over the shelf of Buddhist texts.

Waking up in the morning, the seagulls screech loudly, but I don't mind. I want this time to last forever.

Chapter 7

2015

I'm inside a plastic coffin. My entire self is encased by the whole-body MRI scanner. In one hand, I hold a button which the nurse has told me to press if it all gets too much and I want to stop the scan. Although I'm frightened and claustrophobic, I don't press the button because I know if I stop the scan now, they'll open the machine and I'll breathe for a minute or so, but then they'll start the procedure again from the beginning. The scan takes forty-five minutes and I'm having it because a suspicious shadow showed up on my spine in the last lot of images, which needs further investigation in case it's cancer. I don't want bone metastasis: if the Kraken has extended his tentacles into my bones, I won't be able to lift weights and that will be Bad News. Lungs, spine, then brain is breast cancer's preferred trajectory and I know it's in my lungs now so it would make sense that it's made it to my spine.

I'm experiencing a hot flush. I've been having these since chemotherapy: I feel boiling hot and break out in sweat all over. It's also a side effect of the menopause-inducing treatments: Zoladex and letrazole. Inside the plastic machine it's unbearable. Starting to panic, I almost press the button but stop myself just in time. I don't know how long I've been in here. My dress is stuck to my body with sweat, all I can see is plastic. I can hear the creaking and whirring of the machine.

The coffin is nailed down, I can't lift an arm to break free. *This is what premature burial must feel like*, I think. I read "The Premature Burial" when I was nine. It was in my Edgar Allen Poe collection, illustrated by Gustave Dore, which my Grandad gave me. He marked the scariest stories not to read, so of course I read them first.

The scan seems interminable but at last it ends: the longest fifty minutes of my life. The machine opens, and I climb out.

"How was it?" Dad asks when I find him in the waiting room.

"Terrible," I say. "Like a premature burial."

We walk back to the car through the back streets of Watford. Now to wait for the results and see whether or not I have cancer in my spine.

A couple of weeks later, we're in my oncologist's office for the results.

"Good news," he says, smiling at me. "It's just an overgrown bit of bone on your spine: probably from all that weightlifting you do. It's not cancer."

"Phew," I say, feeling enormous relief: this is the first time in my cancer journey that the worst thing hasn't happened, the first small reprieve. For once we leave the Breast Care Clinic without the worst possible news.

It's mid-May: my birthday is on the fifteenth. Seb comes down on the Thursday and my actual birthday is on the Saturday.

"I've planned a lovely day for you," he says when he arrives. "I was up late last night, I couldn't sleep because I was so excited."

"How lovely," I say, putting my arms round him, gazing into his eyes. *I'm so lucky*, I think. Not only is Seb my boyfriend but he's planned a special birthday for me.

"First of all, this," Seb says, handing me a box. Opening it, I find a gold bangle with flower shapes pressed onto it. "The gold will gradually rub off," Seb says. "It's silver underneath. It's the most expensive present I've ever got anybody," he says. "Not that that's the point but it's from a special shop in Brighton and …"

"I love it, darling," I say. "Thank you." Kissing Seb, I put the bracelet on my left wrist. "I will always wear it," I tell him.

We go to the Everyman cinema in Belsize Park to see *The Clouds of Sils Maria,* starring Juliette Binoche and Kristen Stewart. We sit on a sofa and drink champagne. After the film we walk around Belsize Park and down to where Seb's drama school used to be. It's now an art gallery so we wander around there, holding hands. I'm wearing a new dress: long with applique stripes: a sequined rainbow.

Seb has booked at Manna, the posh vegetarian restaurant in Primrose Hill where all the celebrities go, for dinner. We've been here together before: the last time we were together, four years previously, before Seb disappeared into the monastery for three years. This time it's different though. Now we're in a real relationship where Seb returns my feelings, where he buys me jewellery and plans a birthday treat for me.

"I'm so happy, darling," I tell him as we sip our wine.

"Me too," Seb says, gazing at me. I drown in his turquoise eyes. No one else has eyes this colour. "It's all an amazing surprise to be with you, in a relationship, but I'm happy too."

Seb rushes off to stay with his dad the next day. I'm having a party with my chums and he doesn't like large gatherings. I meet my friends at The Engineer gastropub in Primrose Hill and we sit outside. My brother is there and my cousins and all my friends: we sit at tables outside and two of my friends turn up with their Cavalier King Charles spaniel, Blenheim, so called because he's a Blenheim spaniel– chestnut and white.

"I brought Hero and Blenheim because I knew you'd want to see them," my beautiful friend Phoebe says.

"Of course I do," I say, hugging Hero and Blenheim. The last time I was with these girls in Notting Hill we were in a café. Rufus Sewell, the actor, was there and he talked to us, probably because my friends are stunning dog-owning models. I can't now remember what he said but it was very exciting, and he was lovely and looks just like he does on the television.

"Why don't you come round tomorrow afternoon and meet Seb?" I say to Suzy my best friend.

"OK, I will," she says. "Oohhhh I can't believe I'm finally going to be allowed to meet him." She hugs me.

The next day, Seb returns. Suzy comes round with my present, a special book with moving pictures of African animals. She and Seb seem to get on well.

"He's really gorgeous," she says, as she's leaving, smiling at me.

"Of course he is," I say. "Why do you think I like him so much?"

I'm at Seb's mum's house with him. She lives in a beautiful farmhouse set in rolling fields in the South Downs. We're on safari here: it's hot and all the cats and dogs are passed out on the floor. I sit next to Seb on the sofa and Kitty and Wellington, the Ragdolls, Spitfire's Mum and Uncle, lie in fluffy heaps just like wild lions. I'm so happy to be here, with Seb, as his girlfriend at last – eleven years since we met.

It's after dinner. "Can we take a cat up with us?" I ask.

"Let's take the Count," Seb says, which is what he and his brother call Wellington. Picking up the biggest, fluffiest cat, we say our goodnights to Seb's mum and stepdad and climb the stairs to the room we're sleeping in. Sliding under the covers, Seb puts Wellington down on top of us. He's such a beautiful cat: big blue eyes, cream fur with a big ruff round his neck, grey face. He's so soft and such a lovely, gentle person. He loves being brushed: I've got his cream fluff all over my secret support top and pants. A secret support top is a vest top with sewn-in soft bra pads, so it seems like I'm wearing a bra under my top. Wellington has had enough cuddles and stalks off downstairs. Sinking into the deep mattress – "This is too soft, don't you think?" Seb says, I fall asleep with my love.

Waking up the next morning, we drive to Arundel. We have an English breakfast in a little tea shop where all the décor is white. Next door there's an antique prints shop and I buy a couple of prints from *The Tale of Squirrel Nutkin* – one for me and one for Mum. We visit the beautiful church with the amazing rose window and buy post cards. There's a wonderful castle hewn out of the rock, but it's closed today because it's Monday.

"That's a relief," Seb says, as we get back in the car. "I'm too tired to walk round the castle."

"Yeah, me too," I say, putting my hand on his thigh.

We drive back to Worthing where we visit our favourite Turkish restaurant and watch *Peep Show*. Seb has a double bed on the floor, and I lie in it and read Peter Ackroyd's brilliant Hitchcock biography.

"There's something I want to do," Seb says the next morning when we wake up to the screeching of the seagulls.

"What is it, darling?" I ask.

"Well, I've got these folding chairs," he says. "I want to go to Marks and Spencer and buy a picnic and eat it on the beach and …"

"Let's do it," I say. "Can we just have some coffee and …"

"I'll put the kettle on," Seb says. "Do you want a tea or coffee?"

"Coffee please," I say, smiling at my love.

We walk along the sea front towards Marks and Spencer. Once we're there, we buy salads and sandwiches and crisps and olives and a bottle of white wine. I love the Worthing Marks and Spencer. Seb does most of his shopping here: he's never quite learnt to economise, the dear sweet boy. We pay for our purchases and walk back along the sea front, across the pebbles at the top of the beach and down to the sand. I'm carrying the shopping and Seb is carrying the chairs. Putting them down on the sand, he opens them out: they're metal poles encased in fabric for the bodies of the chairs.

"I've wanted to do this for ages," Seb says. "I've been driving around with these chairs in my car, wanting to have a picnic but it's never been the right time."

"And now it is," I say, sitting in my chair. The wine glasses we've bought are too big to fit in the cup holders on the arms of the chairs, so I rest mine on the sand, hoping it doesn't fall over.

Seb pours me a glass of wine. I drink it, and then another. Starting to feel a bit drunk, I realise I'm crying. Clambering onto Seb's lap, I cry into his hair.

"What is it?" Seb asks.

"I love you," I say. "I want to get married and …"

"We've been through this before," Seb says, sounding resigned. "You know I don't want to get married so …"

"But I do," I say, through my tears. "I want to get married before I die, and I love you and I want to spend the rest of my life with you and …"

"Look," Seb says, stroking my arm. "I'm happy with you now, in the moment. It feels right, now. I can't make any promises about the future or …"

"I know," I say, gulping back my tears. "I'm sorry, darling." *You said you'd stay with me until the end*, I think.

Sitting on Seb's lap, wrapped in his strong arms, I look out to a sea which is the turquoise of Seb's eyes. We have the beach to ourselves. A couple of seagulls sit next to us on the sand. I want this time to last forever: I'm happy here with Seb, in Worthing, this summer after his exams. In September he'll attend university and everything will be different. I've grown fond of Seb's studio flat in this sleepy seaside town. I love the beach here. I love our Turkish restaurant and we've been so happy here since my first visit with my cousins back in March. I'm scared of change. I'm scared our relationship won't survive when he goes to university. And now I'm crying again.

"What is it?" Seb asks, kissing my forehead. "What's the matter?"

"We've been so happy here," I say, looking out to sea. "I'm scared everything is going to change when you go to university."

"You can visit me in Exeter," he says. "It's really beautiful coastline there – much more beautiful than here."

"OK," I say, feeling my tears dry up. "OK, I will." But the niggling feeling everything is about to change, that this is the high point of our relationship and it's all downhill from here persists, much as I try to ignore it.

Chapter 8

2016

"Let's just film that again," the director says. We're at my gym, we've hired a whole studio here and a film crew are filming my personal training session with my Spanish trainer Katharina. "Just do that sequence again please."

Picking up the baguette-shaped weighted bag, Katharina places it on my shoulders.

"Hold the straps at the front," she says in her Valencian accent, smiling at me. "That's right. Now do lunges down the length of the room."

Dipping, I drop my back knee to the floor, stand up, dip the alternate knee, put one foot in front of the other and drop the back knee and repeat until I've crossed the whole length of the wooden floor.

"Very good," the director says in his Glaswegian burr. "Did you catch that?" He asks the cameraman.

"Yes, it's all good," the cameraman says.

Ten years before – back in 2006 – I'd appeared on a BBC2 programme called *The Secret Life of the Manic Depressive,* presented by Stephen Fry. Now, ten years on, the commissioner of the programme, now promoted to BBC1, is doing a follow-up programme to see how Stephen is faring now. The director found me through my blog, and they're filming me at a personal training session, as exercise is what keeps me well.

"Get that step," the director says. "Let's film a bit of weightlifting."

Katharina fetches the plastic step and I lie on top of it. She hands me the twenty kg. bar, and I lift it, up and back down to my chest. The cameras roll. There are five of them: three cameramen, the director and an assistant who makes all the arrangements. One of the cameramen seems to be filming into my crotch to get the right angle as I lift the bar up, then down. Gazing up at the ceiling, I see dust on top of the long strip lights that hang down. I'm wearing a full face of make-up, which I never wear for training, and my fluorescent orange top, multi-coloured patterned shorts and purple trainers. My hair is loose to look better on film.

"Let's just try that again, from the other side," the director says, and the cameraman moves then films me lifting the weight up and down, up and down.

We're at the hospital. I'm sitting next to Mum, outside in the corridor in radiography, waiting for a CT scan. My film crew are with me.

"Talk about something," the director says. The cameramen are seated with their backs against one wall, then there's us, then the corner and round the corner are an elderly couple no doubt waiting for a scan. *They must wonder who we are and what we're doing*, I think, looking at them. Maybe they assume we're filming a hospital drama – *Casualty* or *Holby City*. I bet they think I'm some annoying actress. They won't have any idea I'm a bipolar patient with secondary breast cancer, waiting for a scan to see if the cancer in my lungs has spread.

"So here we are in the hospital of death and cancer," I say.

"Just keep talking," the director says, looking at me and Mum. Resting my head on Mum's shoulder for a moment, I close my eyes. I'm so tired.

"Roger and Rafa are both still in," Mum says, looking animated as she starts to talk about the French Open tennis that is happening at the moment. "Do you think either of them could win it or …"

"What about Andy or Novak?" I say.

"Well, Rafa's pretty much unbeatable on clay," Mum says.

"It would be amazing if Andy won," I say.

"He won't though," Mum says, shaking her head. "Rafa's going to win again I should think and ..."

"OK, that's enough," the director says. "I didn't say 'talk about the bloody tennis', I mean you two – what are you like?" He sighs.

"Right, if you keep drinking that water," a nurse says, bustling up to me. "You're going in for your scan next and I want you to have drunk a litre of water."

"Oh, OK, sorry," I say, pouring myself a plastic cup of water, downing it, then pouring another one.

"It's time now," the nurse says, taking me into the room with the scanner. "You'll have to film through the window, I'm afraid," she says to my film crew. "You're not allowed in the room because of the patient's privacy."

Inside the room, I lie back on the bed. A nurse comes over with a cannula to insert into my left arm: they have to use this as I've had all the nodes out on my right side. I can't have injections there due to the risk of lymphoedema – my whole arm will swell up. This isn't just a one-off event either – once you've had lymphoedema it keeps coming back. It's a serious problem – just one of the many nasty things breast cancer throws at you.

"Are you alright, love?" she asks, looking concerned.

"Yes, it's just my film crew are here," I say. "They're filming a programme about my mental disorder for BBC1 and ... ouch ... " I say as the cannula goes into the back of my hand.

"So, this scan is the one where you'll feel like you're wetting yourself, but you're not," the nurse says. "We're going to do it now."

Lying back on the bed, I feel so sorry for myself. Here I am, having yet another scan to see if the cancer has spread from my lungs and there's a film crew here. I can't even be alone for this, which ought to be a private time. This is, of course, my own fault. When the film crew asked if they could come to the hospital, I could have said no, but to be honest I just assumed the NHS wouldn't let them film here. I was wrong. There's even a media officer at the hospital whose job it is to make sure the day goes without a hitch. She's with us today, of course.

Tears roll down my cheeks. Opening my eyes, I see the crew filming me crying.

The scanning machine is a big white polo mint: a round machine with a large hole in the middle where the bed goes. The machine will travel up and down the bed, scanning. The nurses leave the room and I'm on my own. Whirring, the machine moves down the bed, over my chest, collecting its pictures. I feel a hot flush rush through my body and then a peculiar sensation: I'm wetting myself. Then it passes.

"Very good," the nurse says, coming back into the room. "I'll just take the cannula out of your hand and then you can go home."

"Thank you," I say, as she removes the cannula from my hand and puts a plaster over the little hole. I haven't wet myself, I realise.

We walk back to our various cars in the hospital car park and the film crew follow us to my parental home. When we arrive, Spitfire is sitting on the doorstep.

"Hello Fluffy Monster," I say, picking him up. "Can Spitfire be in the film?" I ask the director, carrying my giant cat down the stairs.

"OK, if you sit on the stairs with the cat on your lap," the director says.

Sitting on the stairs, I place Spitfire on my lap. I'm wearing a navy dress and as I stroke him, he deposits orange fur on my lap.

"So, Spitfire is my cat, Seb's mum's cat's kitten" I say to the director. "But he lives here because when we got him, I was having chemotherapy and I wasn't well enough to look after him, but now Mum won't let him live in my flat with me and …"

"You couldn't look after him," Mum says. "And you're here too much of the time anyway, with all your medical appointments and …"

"But he's my cat," I say, feeling sad. "I want him to live with me."

"You can visit him here as often as you want," Mum says.

Stroking my Precious Angel Fluffball, he feels so soft. Ragdolls were bred to have silky fur and he's inherited this from his Mum. He's also inherited her short legs and separation anxiety – he can't stand to be shut in a room away from us. When he was a baby, he pulled up the carpet in his bedroom, shutting himself in by mistake. Now he sleeps on top of my parents in their bedroom every night.

"Right, I'm just going to interview your mum for a bit, that was great," the director says. Spitfire climbs down from my lap and stalks away, heading for the garden.

We're at the zoo. This is the last bit of filming and I'm here with Mum and the young cameraman, just the three of us. In the time since the scan my mood has crashed. The panther stalks around next to me. He is always with me at the moment.

We're at Penguin Beach. It's a large pool, where the penguins swim. There are Perspex sections where you can watch them underwater. We walk across the front of the pool, watching penguins swimming in front of us. There is a sheet of Perspex almost as tall as me so we can see the penguins somersaulting in the water.

At the side of the main pool, there is a nursery one where the chicks live. There are a couple of very new ones who are grey and fluffy.

"Hello little chap," I say, bending down to look a penguin chick in the eye.

"Isn't he a dolly?" Mum says, putting her arm round me. "Hello sweetie," she says to him. The chicks waddle over to us, across the concrete. Up the steps I can see our cameraman filming us with the chicks.

"Let's go and film with the pelicans and flamingos," he says, picking up his camera. It's on a big tripod and he struggles to carry the whole thing. He's a lovely guy: he's about thirty, blond and very chilled and kind.

The flamingos and pelicans live on an island just round the corner from Penguin Beach and we head for it, taking the path, the panther bounding along next to us.

Leaning on the railings, I look at the pelicans and flamingos. There's grass in front of me and some of the pelicans waddle across the grass: huge beaks jutting out in front of them. They're massive cream-coloured birds with big dark eyes. Behind these few pelicans there's water, and across the water there's an island where the flock of flamingos stand, on one leg: bright coral pink ballerinas. Some bend long necks and dip their curved bills into the water, sifting it for shrimps. There are a few chicks on the island, and they are grey with sticking-out feathers and long legs.

"OK, that's great," the cameraman says. "Let's go to the other side of the zoo and see the giraffes now."

"Do you want some help carrying that camera?" Mum asks.

"No, it's fine, I can manage," he says, smiling at Mum.

We walk through the tunnel to the other side of the zoo. I am tired: my legs are aching and I just want to go home. With my depression, I feel a terrible physical sensation of the whole world pressing down on me and time passes so slowly. The panther pushes into me, reminding me of his presence: as if I could ever forget.

"I want to go home," I say to Mum.

"Just this last bit, darling," Mum says, putting her arm round me. "You want to see the giraffes before we go don't you?"

"Yes, I suppose so," I say. I do want to see them but my legs and back hurt from all the walking and I just want to go to bed – I've missed my afternoon sleep to do this filming and with my mood this low, I'm exhausted.

At last, we're at the Giraffe House. Leaning on the fence, I watch a giraffe as she eats some browse, her jaw chomping the branch with that side-to-side action. She sticks out a long blue tongue to pull the leaves into her mouth. The panther is scared of giraffes: he crouches down, flat to the ground.

"So, how do you feel now?" the cameraman asks me, filming me.

"Now, my mood is low and I'm so tired," I say. "I'm trudging through treacle and the sky's pressing down on me, and I don't want to be here, even though this is my happy place and … "

"You're doing really well," he says. "We've filmed some other people when they're depressed and they can't do anything and here *you* are, having a day out and enjoying yourself and … "

"I push myself," I say, looking at the yellow and brown diamond pattern on the Rothschild giraffe's neck as she bends her head to eat. "I've had this illness all my adult life – I've had to learn to cope with it."

The panther stands next to me, watching the giraffe. *I bet he'd like to sink his teeth into her flank*, I think.

"OK, I think I've got enough footage now," the cameraman says, putting his camera away. "Thank you very much, ladies."

"Thank you," I say, feeling relieved it's over and we can go home, and I can lie down.

"Will you be alright getting home with that huge thing?" Mum asks him, looking concerned.

"Yes, fine," he says. "I think we got some good stuff today." He smiles at us.

Chapter 9

2015

Waking up with a jolt, I focus slowly. I'm in hospital: I've just had a skin-sparing mastectomy on my left side. I have three drains and my whole chest is wrapped in plastic tape. I can tell I will be allergic to this one: as I am to all the plastic dressings, to everything except pink Micropore tape and Elastoplast. Checking my clock, I see it's six o'clock in the morning. Ah. Early. My mood is up and the morphine and operation have sent it further up. I'm in severe pain in my chest. Ringing my bell, I wait for a nurse to answer.

My door opens. A nurse bustles in.

"How can I help you?" she asks, looking at me.

"So, I'm in a lot of pain," I say, the words rushing out of my mouth at speed, tumbling over each other. "So please can I have some morphine and …"

She picks up my drug chart which is on the table under my television on the other side of the room and examines it. "Yes, I'll get you some," she says.

"Thank you," I say, glad that pain relief is coming.

She leaves the room.

Pressing the control attached to my bedside table, I raise the upper section of my bed so I'm sitting up. I love this about the hospital bed.

I haven't slept well because, as I've had surgery on my chest, I've had to sleep on my back rather than on my front which I am used to. Also, my high mood wakes me at six o'clock in the morning. Plus, there's the pain in my chest.

The nurse returns with a tiny paper cup of Oramorph. Downing the sweet liquid, I take the two ibuprofen as well, and the big antibiotic pill, which is to ensure my wounds don't become infected.

"Let's just do your blood pressure," the nurse says, wheeling the machine over to my bed. I stick out my finger and she clamps it in the device. I have to have my blood pressure taken like this, again because I've had all my nodes removed from under both arms. She puts the band round my calf instead, fastening the Velcro so it's tight. It hurts.

"Very good," she says, looking at the numbers on the screen.

"Is my blood pressure OK?" I ask.

"Yes, it's perfect," she says.

"Can you help me go to the loo please?" I ask.

"OK, let's unclip these drain bottles," she says. The bottles are clipped onto the sides of my bed, to make sure I don't get tangled up in their tubes in the night.

Leaning on the nurse, I step out of bed and onto the floor, wobbling. I hold my drain bottles and their tubes in a plastic bag. It's just a few steps to the bathroom and it's a relief to sit on the loo. Doing a wee, wiping my bottom, I get up and step over to the sink to wash my hands, still carrying my bottles.

"Let's get you back in bed then," the nurse says, helping me across the room and back into bed, clipping the bottles to either side of my bed.

"My chest hurts," I say.

"The morphine will start to work soon," she says, wheeling the blood pressure machine out, closing my door.

I'm alone again. I don't want to be alone. I want my mum. It's only 6.15 a.m. so I can't phone Mum yet. I'm watching *Breaking Bad,* so I turn my television on and become absorbed by Walter and Jesse's escapades.

But I can't concentrate because my mood is too high. Pressing the pantry button, I wait for attention.

"Yes?" someone answers.

"Can I have some coffee please?" I ask.

"Coming up," the voice says.

A few minutes later, there's a knock on my door.

"Come in," I say.

"Here's your coffee," the waitress says. She wears a black trouser suit with a white pinny tied in front of it.

"Thank you," I say.

She pushes the special table over my bed so I can drink my coffee. I pour it into the cup and take a sip.

I'm trying to watch *Breaking Bad*, but I can't concentrate. My thoughts are racing. Now I need the loo again. Pushing the table away, I put my drain bottles back into the plastic bag and shuffle on wobbling legs to the bathroom. All this coffee isn't going to stop my anxiety, it's going to make it worse, but with my high mood I just want to elevate it further – that's one of the things about hypomania, the brain's desire to build on it and to send your mood up and up.

At last, it's seven o'clock and I can phone my parents.

"Hello?" Mum answers the phone.

"Mum, can you come and see me please?" I ask, my words tumbling out.

"Hello, darling," Mum says. "I'll come and see you in about an hour and … "

"Why can't you come now?" I ask.

67

"Because I've only just woken up – I've got to feed your cat and have a bath and get dressed," Mum says. "Stop talking so fast, your speech sounds pressured."

"I'm not speaking fast and the nurses aren't giving me enough attention," I say.

"They have to look after all the other patients too," Mum says. "Stop that pressured speech. I'll see you in about an hour and … "

"I love you Mum," I say, trying to keep the desperation out of my voice. I don't want to be on my own.

"I love you too, darling," Mum says. "Try to calm down."

I'm not calm so I drink more coffee and my mood rises further.

At long last Mum arrives and she sits with me whilst I talk rubbish and then we watch some *Top Gear* and Mum helps me to the loo.

"Why don't you read some of your book, darling?" Mum says when she's trying to leave.

"Can't concentrate," I say. "My chest hurts."

"It isn't time for your morphine yet," Mum says.

Mum goes home and I cry because I don't want to be on my own.

Pressing the nurse call button, I wait for some attention. I just want someone to come and talk to me. Dad won't be here till this evening which is many hours away still.

There's a knock at my door.

"Come in," I say.

A nurse opens the door. "How are you?" she asks. She's an older lady, this one. Haven't seen her before.

"Is it time for me to have some more Oramorph?" I ask.

"Let me just check your chart," she says. Picking my drug chart up from the table under the television, she examines it. "Yes, I can give you some Oramorph," she says. "I'll just go and get that and your antibiotic and then we can do your blood pressure."

"Thank you," I say. "I'm quite anxious, I'm just wondering if I can have some clonazepam or lorazepam or diazepam or something like that?"

"We're not authorised to give you that," she says. "I'll have to ask a pharmacist."

"Oh," I say. "Would you be able to help me have a bath?"

"You mustn't get the dressings wet," she says, looking at my chest. "I suppose you can sit in the bath and wash your legs and lower body."

"Yes please," I say.

Taking the hospital gown off, I can see the tight plastic wrapping all around my chest. It's so uncomfortable. I have no idea what my skin looks like underneath and I don't want to find out. Hobbling into the bathroom, carrying my drain bottles in a plastic bag, I sit in the bath and turn the taps on. The sound of running water soothes me.

"I thought you might not be allowed real flowers, so I brought you these," Seb says, handing me a bouquet of peach fabric roses.

"Thank you, darling," I say. It's Friday night and he's come to visit me in hospital.

We watch *A Lion Called Christian* and the Michael Sheen film *The Damned United*. I loved the David Peace book so much. When I lived in West Hampstead I had a poster for the film, but I left it there when I moved out, which is sad.

I'm so happy he's come to see me in hospital.

"I love you, darling," I say to him.

"My feelings for you fluctuate," he says.

"Can't you even say you love me when I'm in hospital and I've just had major surgery?" I say.

"My feelings fluctuate," he says. "They're not stable and ..."

"I think you'd better go," I say, scratching at my plastic bandages which have started to make me itch like crazy. I feel so cross with Seb.

He can't even tell me he loves me when I've just had an operation. I don't want him here. "Just go," I say.

"OK, I'll call you tomorrow," he says, shutting the door behind him.

When he's gone I burst into tears and pull all my bandages off. I have come up in a rash under them and I scratch my burning skin.

"So, how are you?" my psychiatrist Dr Stein asks, sitting in a chair next to my bed. His blue eyes are full of concern. It's Saturday morning and I had my operation on Tuesday. He works at this hospital today so he's popped in to see how I'm getting on.

"Well, I'm very anxious," I say. "And I asked if I could have some clonazepam and the nurses said no and … "

"Your mood is very elevated," he says. "I don't know why the hospital didn't call me and ask me to come and see you days ago."

"I don't know," I say. "I've been telling the nurses that I'm very anxious for days and …"

"Well, never mind," he says. "I'm here now. I'll speak to the pharmacist and make sure they prescribe you some clonazepam – we need to get your mood down to a manageable level and …"

"Thank you so much," I say, smiling at him. *Some clonazepam is coming*, I think. *This terrible anxiety is going to be dealt with.*

"Well, Seb came to see me yesterday," I say. "And he said his feelings for me fluctuate and …." I'm crying. "If he doesn't love me, what's the point?" I ask, through gasping sobs.

"Now, you're just upset because your mood is too high and you had an argument with your boyfriend," Dr Stein says, patting my hand. "I'll get you the clonazepam and within thirty minutes or so you should feel calmer. It's very bad that they didn't contact me days ago: it's lucky I'm here now."

"Thank you," I say.

"I'll see you soon," he says, getting up to go.

A nurse brings the clonazepam, I take it, and about forty minutes later my anxiety subsides a bit. My mood is still elevated, and I don't help it by ordering coffee all the time.

Dad comes to see me in the evening, and we watch a film whilst I eat my supper: omelette and toast. I'm allowed a glass of red wine and that helps me calm down a bit. Dad too is a calming presence and I'm starting to feel better – the clonazepam is working. Dad has brought me some avocado, cut up by Mum, and I eat whilst we watch Hitchcock's film of Somerset Maugham's *Ashenden*. It's a black-and-white film called *Secret Agent* and stars John Gielgud, Madeleine Carroll and Peter Lorre. John Gielgud plays Ashenden, an English spy in the First World War. It's set in Switzerland and as the characters climb mountains, and Ashenden tries to stop an enemy agent carrying out his mission, I focus on the film and start to feel calmer. When Dad leaves after the film, I turn my light out and after taking my night-time meds, I do my body scan meditation. *Things will be OK with Seb*, I think. *I was just upset*. Closing my eyes, I drift into sleep.

Chapter 10

I'm on all fours, in front of the television, vomiting into a bucket. *Gone With the Wind* is playing: it's nearly Christmas, and even though I'm throwing my guts up, I refuse to miss my favourite film. More vomit comes up. I don't know where it's all coming from. My throat and tummy feel very sore. I was just released from hospital the day before: Mum made them take my drains out: "I'm not having you home with drains in," she said.

Atlanta is burning and Scarlett is sitting up at the front of the wagon with Rhett whilst Melanie and the baby are in the back. Flames engulf the screen. Another wave of nausea hits me and I'm being sick into my bucket again. This is horrible: tears of distress run down my cheeks. I think I'm going to have to give up on the film after all and go back to bed. I don't know why I'm so nauseous but I need to go back to bed. Picking up my bucket, I shuffle through the house to my bedroom, head spinning.

The next day, I'm at the farm with Mum. Whatever was making me sick has passed: I realise that it was the now-empty bottle of Oramorph which I hid from Mum when I was discharged from hospital. Bad me. It was nice though, apart from the puking. Now I'm accompanying Mum to the farm shop. We've parked the car and I notice a barn which I've never seen before.

"Look Mum," I say, looking at the door of the barn. "It's a Spin studio. I can come to classes here and …"

"Please, have one of these," an Italian man in cycling gear says. "Here's a timetable, come back and try a class."

"Thank you," I say, looking at the timetable. "I'll come back tomorrow."

"Very good. You won't be disappointed," he says, smiling at me. "I'm Giorgio, I run this place – it's called Cyclezone."

"Have you been open long?" I ask.

"About one year," he says.

"Well, I'm going to be staying with my parents for a while whilst I recover from an operation, so this is perfect," I say. "I was at Virgin Active in Borehamwood but they closed down and …"

"Ah, I used to teach at Virgin, back in the day," he says. "Come back tomorrow, nine thirty in the morning," he says. "I'll see you then."

"Thank you, I will," I say, smiling at him.

"Well, that's a piece of luck," Mum says.

As we drive out of the farm, we see a couple of horses in the field: a chestnut and a palomino. They're chomping the grass but lift their heads to look at us as we drive off.

The next morning, I'm awake early – my mood is still up. Putting a sports bra over my cosmetic surgery bra and a vest top over that, I pull on some trousers and trainers, and a long-sleeved top over my vest top.

"Come on, it's nine o'clock," Mum says. "We'd better get going"

"I'm ready," I say, picking up a fabric bag with a bottle of water, waiting by the front door for Mum to open it.

Arriving at the farm, we get out of the car and head towards the barn. Opening the glass door, I see a room of Spin bikes and a clock on one wall made from a bike wheel with hands stuck on top.

"Ah, hello ladies," Giorgio says. "Find a bike and I'll be with you in a moment to help you set up."

"I'll be back for you in forty-five minutes," Mum says, stroking my arm. "Be careful: don't push yourself too hard."

"I will," I say. "I mean, I won't."

I choose a bike at the far left-hand side of a row, as the walls are all mirrored and I'll be able to see my position. Also, I won't have to have anyone on one side of me, which is good. Filling up my water bottle, I put it in the indent on one side of the handlebars and tuck the bottoms of my trousers into my socks.

"Right, any illnesses or injuries I should know about?" the instructor asks. She's pretty with long, dark hair in a ponytail. "My name is Heather for those who don't know me and …"

"I've just had chest surgery," I say. "But the doctors say it's fine for me to do this."

"OK, well, be careful and take it easy," she says. "Let's have some music and get going then, everyone."

She switches on the speaker and climbs onto her bike which faces the class.

"Right, everybody, I want you to put a bit of resistance on," she says. "So that's gear three or four on your monitor. Turn the red dial in front of you to the right."

I feel my pedals becoming harder to push round.

"This is just the warm-up," she says. "Don't put too much resistance on yet."

The lights are dimmed and now there are blue ones and coloured ones flashing down from the timbers of the barn.

"Standing flat," Heather says. "Stand up on your pedals and rest your hands in front of you, take the weight on your legs, don't lean on your arms, that's right."

"Accelerate," Heather says, running as she stands up.

It's easier to move the pedals round from standing, so I can run on my pedals too.

"Take a seat everyone, take a drink and turn your resistance down. Let's take a recovery," Heather says.

Throughout all of this the lights are flashing and there's pumping dance music playing. Taking a gulp of my water, wiping the sweat from my forehead with my towel, I think how much I'm enjoying myself. I've been to Spin classes before but there's something about the mechanical feel of the bikes and the way the movement blends with the music that makes this class a cut above any other Spin class I've experienced.

"OK, recovery over, we're going to climb," Heather says. "Turn your red dial to the right, I want it to feel heavy. It should be an effort to turn your legs."

It does indeed feel hard to turn my legs.

"Stand up – hands at the top of your handlebars," she says, standing up and moving her hands right to the ends of her handlebars. "Nice arch in your back – we're climbing."

Copying her, I stand up, slide my hands to the ends of the handlebars and feel the climb become easier. Turning my red dial to the right a bit more, I make the climb more intense.

There are about fourteen girls, including me, and two men. Giorgio, the chap we met yesterday, is sitting at a desk at the back of the room, answering messages on his phone and fiddling with his iPad.

"Turn it up," Heather says. "I want you to get out of your comfort zone and challenge yourself. This is your ride: have you got any more to give? You might already be working at your limit, but if you're not, turn it up."

Turning my resistance up, I see it hit number six. It's tough, climbing this hill, but I feel great.

"Combinations," Heather says. "Four up, four down. One, two, three, four – now stand up. One, two, three, four – now sit down. Excellent. Keep going."

"Stay high," she says. "Add a bit of resistance."

I settle into a rhythm for the standing climb. This is easier than sitting so I add a bit more resistance.

"Ninety seconds," Heather says. "Recovery is coming up. You're doing really well everyone."

I realise I'm running out of water, so I get down from my bike, quickly refill my water bottle and climb back onto my bike, just as everyone is sitting down for recovery. Taking a bit of resistance off, sipping my water, I feel pleased with myself. I've only been out of hospital for a couple of days but I'm in a Spin class and keeping up.

"Right, we're going to sprint," Heather says. "It's a flat road, so take some resistance off, but I want you to speed up to ninety RPM, no more than a hundred."

Turning my red dial to the left, moving my legs faster, I get my pace up to about eighty. Taking a bit more resistance off, I hit ninety.

"I want you to keep your pace at ninety and add a tweak of resistance," Heather says. Adding a tweak to the right, I push harder but my pace drops down to eighty-five. Turning my resistance down a bit, I get my pace back up to ninety. *I'm doing really well*, I think. This is my first class after all.

"Keep going," Heather says. "Accelerate, accelerate."

Her legs are spinning round so fast. I try to copy her, but I can't quite get my speed up. I take a sip of water.

"OK everyone," Heather says. "Turn your dial all the way to the left. That's it. Breathe in through the nose for three and out through the mouth for five, that will get your heart rate back down. When you're ready, stop cycling."

She guides us through some stretches: the first few on the bike followed by calf, glute and hamstring stretches off the bike.

"How did you find the class?" Giorgio asks me afterwards.

"Brilliant, I loved it," I say, wiping down my handlebars with a wet wipe and rubbing them with a towel. "I'm going to come back every day."

"Excellent," he says, smiling. "Glad you enjoyed it."

"Thank you, Giorgio, thank you Heather," I say, putting my long-sleeved top on. "See you tomorrow."

"See you tomorrow, sweetheart," she says, smiling at me.

Opening the glass door, I step outside the barn to wait for Mum, smiling that I've had such a great time at the class.

Chapter 11

"Hello, my darling," I say, opening the door of the flat to see Seb standing there, huge rucksack over one shoulder. He always brings his pillow plus some clothes plus who-knows-what-else in this huge rugby bag.

"Hello, my lovely," Seb drawls. Putting our arms around each other, we embrace and have a snog.

I'm wearing my high-heeled, black rubber Melissa shoes with the flowers on the heels. Clop, clop, clopping down the hallway to the lounge, Seb follows me, putting his enormous bag down on the floor.

"Would you like a drink, my darling?" I ask.

"An Old Fashioned," Seb says, smiling at me. We've just started watching *Mad Men* and it's Don Draper's go-to drink. "I've brought the ingredients, I'll make it myself. You?"

"Gin and Slimline tonic, please," I say.

"One gin and Slimline tonic coming up," Seb says, taking a bottle of gin from the kitchen countertop, pouring an inch into a glass, adding ice, squeezing a piece of lime into it, filling the glass with Slimline tonic.

"Thank you, darling," I say, taking the drink from him, sitting in the nest in front of the television, watching him make his drink. He places a sugar cube in a glass and saturates it with angostura bitters, adding a dash of plain water. He muddles it till the sugar dissolves.

Filling the glass with ice cubes, he adds whisky and garnishes it with a slice of orange.

Sitting down next to me in the nest, Seb clinks his glass against mine.

"Cheers my lovely," he says, gazing into my eyes.

"Cheers," I say, gazing into his turquoise eyes. *Things seem fine between us*, I think. I'd better not ask him if he loves me though, just in case he says he doesn't, as he did when I was in hospital a mere couple of weeks ago.

"Oh, I brought you a present," he says, putting his drink down on the table, stepping over to his bag.

"I brought you a present too," I say, handing him a package.

We open our presents. Mine is a cotton dressing gown with a seventies-style flowery print in pink, orange, mustard and lilac. "Thank you, darling." I say, kissing him on the cheek – although I feel disappointed he hasn't given me something more romantic, like the bracelet or necklace he gave me last year.

"These are great," Seb says, pulling his gloves from the wrapping. They're grey wool and have a wolf's head on one palm and on the other, a full moon. "I love them, my lovely," he says, kissing me.

"Ah, I'm glad you like them," I say, smiling.

We settle down in the nest to watch *Mad Men* and as we watch the antics of Don Draper and his chums, I feel content. Seb is here: he wants to be with me. He's spending New Year's Eve with me. Things are OK. I'm starting to recover from surgery and I'm in my flat with my boyfriend, having a nice time.

"Are you happy, darling?" I ask, turning towards Seb, resting on my elbow so I can look at him properly.

"Yes, of course I am, my lovely," he says, smiling at me.

Seb returns to Exeter the next day.

January 2016

I decide, rather than a detox, to do Ginuary, which is a commitment to make a different gin cocktail every day of January and to document my creations on Instagram and write about them in my blog. Returning to the parental home, I look at Mum's old book from the seventies, *Cocktails and Mixed Drinks,* and the new book my cousin has just given me, *Tequila Mockingbird,* a book of cocktails inspired by works of literature.

My friend Ben comes to visit on the third of January. We make the Emerald Isle cocktail which is gin, crème de menthe and angostura bitters.

"Not bad," Ben says, sipping his cocktail.

"Ginuary is great," I say, sitting down at the marble table in the parental dining room. "I'm learning all these new and interesting cocktails."

"I like this one," Ben says. "Very green."

Indeed, it's bright green and tastes better than it looks.

"Ben," I say. "I've had a brilliant idea."

"Go on," Ben says, looking at me as he sips his green cocktail.

"So," I say. "I could start writing a new blog, not about dating – I mean I've been with Seb for eleven months now so I'm not dating anyway. The new blog could be about my Spin cycling and it could have these drinks in it and I can call it *The Rapid Cyclist* – because I have the rapid cycling form of bipolar disorder, do you see?"

"Yes, go on," Ben says, looking interested.

"So, it will be a cycling and exercise and sportswear blog," I say. "And it will have about my mental disorder, obviously, and the cancer treatment, and at the moment it will have the gin cocktails every day and …"

"It sounds great," Ben says. "To *The Rapid Cyclist*. The New Year and new beginnings. Cheers," he says.

"Cheers." I say.

I start the new blog that evening and write both of them concurrently for a few days, but soon give up my successful blog, *Scars, Tears and Training Bras*, with its four hundred followers, to concentrate on the new one. *The Rapid Cyclist* is a riot of bright-coloured sportswear, photos of cocktails and, unlike my previous blog, it's not anonymous. I use my real name and have photos of myself at Spin in my new leopard print and tiger print leggings. I still call Spitfire "the Fluffy Monster" but it feels good not to be writing anonymously. Oh, and of course I still call my boyfriend Seb. *It will probably take a while to build up my readership for the new blog*, I think, and invite all the followers of the old blog onto the new blog.

Later, in January, I'm at a flat in Hampstead, sitting on a blanket on top of a white sofa. Next to me, there's a Keeshond – a Spitz breed of dog who looks like a small black, silver and grey long-haired wolf. I call him Mr Fluffypants and I met him through Borrow My Doggy. I read an article by the cat and nature writer Tom Cox about it and decided to join. As soon as I saw there was a Keeshond near me, I messaged his owners and met them – and him. And now here I am, looking after him once a week.

"Shall we go for a walk, Mr Fluffypants?" I ask.

Trotting in front of me, Mr Fluffypants pulls his ears into his head in a process his owners term "streamlining". He's such a good boy – he doesn't pull on the lead at all as we hit Hampstead High Street and head down the hill towards Belsize Park. We pass designer clothes shops, including Question Air where I purchased a couple of Vivienne Westwood Red Label dresses a while back – a black one and a pink one with a large blue print on it.

On our left we pass the Victorian masterpiece of St Stephen's with its French outline – steep roofs and a massive square tower with a big rose window at the front, and ornamental brickwork under the tower and in the transepts in a Moorish style. The church's brick exterior varies from pale grey to Indian red, giving it a mottled appearance. The decorative stone bands are cream-coloured Kentish Rag from Maidstone.

On our right, across the road is the red brick and terracotta marvel that is now Air Studios. Designed by Alfred Waterhouse, who also designed the Natural History Museum in South Kensington, it's a Romanesque style church built on an irregular hexagonal plan with gabled frontages to each side. It's one of my favourite buildings. We pass the town hall and the petrol station and then we're in the middle of Belsize Park. Ahead of us are the cafés and restaurants. We wait to cross the road.

"Sit, Mr Fluffypants," I say.

Mr Fluffypants looks up at me with big brown eyes, his tail curled over his bottom, but doesn't sit.

"Sit!" I say, pointing at the ground. "I know you know how to sit, come on Mr Fluffypants," I say, a pleading note entering my voice. Eventually he sits. Then the lights change, and we cross the road.

Passing the Everyman Cinema and Budgens, we go back past the Old Town Hall and the petrol station, back past Air Studios and St Stephen's. The hill is steeper now, I huff and puff a bit with the effort. It's getting dark now and all the Christmas lights come on – the bare branches of the trees are bedecked with fairy lights. Hampstead looks magical. Turning right just before the kitchen shop, we walk along Willoughby Road and then take a right towards where Mr Fluffypants lives. He bounds up the stairs to the front door of the block. As I open the door, he pushes ahead of me up the stairs and waits for me to open the front door of his flat.

"Here we are, darling," I say, opening the front door of his flat, taking my coat and boots off. Unclipping his harness, I put it back in the basket. He walks over to his water bowl in the kitchen, and I hear him slurping his water.

Chapter 12

2016

Today's cocktail is called a Princeton. The first known recipe for this cocktail was published in George J. Kappeler's 1895 book *Modern American Drinks* where he calls for "A mixing-glass half-full fine ice, three dashes orange bitters, one and a half pony Tom gin. Mix, strain into cocktail-glass; add half a pony port wine carefully and let it settle in bottom of cocktail before serving."

Serve in a Coupe glass. Ingredients: 60ml Tanqueray Old Tom gin, 5ml sugar syrup (two sugar to one water), three dashes of Angostura Orange Bitters, 15ml port. How to make: stir all ingredients with ice and strain into a chilled glass. Garnish with an orange zest twist. Kappeler's 1895 recipe calls for the Old Tom, gin and orange bitters to be stirred with ice and strained into a glass, with tawny port poured down the side of the glass so it settles to form a red layer beneath the orange bitters tinted gin. *Difford's Guide for Discerning Drinkers* adds a spoon (5ml) of sugar syrup to Kappeler's recipe to sweeten the gin and a splash of water to dilute it. They prefer to abandon the original layering and stir all the ingredients together.

Using some of Dad's port, I make the cocktail. The Princeton is just wonderful: one of the stand-out successes of Ginuary. It's a gorgeous deep burgundy colour – almost purple – and tastes rich and sweet. Sipping it, I feel happy to have discovered such a delicacy. I'll definitely make this one again after the end of the month, I decide. As well as tasting sublime, it packs quite a punch, of course.

Seb comes to see me at the flat and we go out to lunch with my cousin Patrick, his wife Julia and their baby boy at Franco Manca, the pizza restaurant in Belsize Park opposite the Everyman cinema.

I'm holding the baby as we're leaving – standing near the exit with my baby cousin looking over my shoulder.

"I didn't recognise you there for a minute," Seb says, as he returns from the loo.

"Come on, let's go," I say, desperate to leave the busy restaurant suddenly and to be on my own with my Seb, at the flat, watching *Mad Men*.

My cousins drive us home in their new car, called Scruffy. We say goodbye to them and then we're on our own in the flat. Suddenly, I feel sad, not exactly that we're not married with a baby, but something along those lines.

"I always feel a bit … why can't we be more like Patrick and Julia?" I ask Seb, as we settle down into the nest.

"Well, they want the same things," Seb says, unlacing his Caterpillar boots. "They're going in the same direction and …"

"We want some of the same things," I say. "We want to be with each other, don't we?"

"Of course we do, my lovely," Seb says. "Do you want a drink?"

"Gin and Slimline tonic please," I say, smiling at him. *I love Seb*, I think. *He's the love of my life and he's here with me and we've been together for almost a year and we have a strong, solid relationship. There's nothing to worry about. There's no point in comparing our relationship to that of my cousins*, I tell myself, turning the television on, putting the DVD into the player.

The *Mad Men* title sequence starts: the brilliant graphic sequence of Don Draper falling towards the ground through the buildings of Madison Avenue, and I concentrate on watching our programme and enjoying the feeling of my big, strong boyfriend lying next to me. Resting my head on his chest, I put my worries to the back of my mind. As Seb likes to say, the important thing is to be in the moment.

We're at a pub in Belsize Park – The Hill on Haverstock Hill. Seb's sister, Katie, is meeting us for a drink. She's very pretty with bright red dyed hair and she's just so cool. She's the one of Seb's three siblings with whom he's closest: Seb is the third of four and Katie's the youngest. There's just a year between them.

I'm drinking a French 75. This cocktail is named after the French seventy-five millimetre light field gun which, due to its portability and rate of fire, was the mainstay of the French army during the First World War.

Standing at the bar, I watch the barman mix my drink. The wall behind the bar is mirrored and many bottles of spirits stand behind the barman.

"One French 75," he says.

"Thank you," I say, taking it outside to sit with Seb and Katie. There are patio heaters on the terrace so we can sit outside even on a January evening.

We have a pleasant evening. I demolish several cocktails.

"I like your sister," I say to Seb afterwards, as we're lying in bed.

"You were on good form, my lovely," Seb says. "Very entertaining."

"Thank you, darling," I say, closing my eyes.

Seb returns to Exeter, and I return to my parentals, Spin and Spitfire. Spin class every day plus the ritual of cocktail hour somehow results in me drinking less than before and I find myself losing weight. I really look forward to making a different gin cocktail every day and to learning about the history of the different drinks, photographing them and documenting them on my Instagram and in the new blog. I'm happy this January with my cocktail project, my exercise routine and my boyfriend. I speak to Seb every day whilst he's away in Exeter.

Far from the grimness of a detox, this January is fun and fabulous. My mood is up, which helps of course, but Spin and Ginuary are important components too.

I'm at Mr Fluffypants' flat. All I have with me to drink is gin and Diet Red Bull, so that's the day's cocktail. I feel that Ginuary has helped me to drink more like a normal person: one glass of wine at lunchtime, one cocktail at six o'clock in the evening and a couple of glasses of wine with dinner. I had been feeling late last year that I was drinking too much with Seb, but now I'm drinking a manageable amount. I stop worrying about having an alcohol problem. After all, I'm functioning. I'm exercising every day and writing every day and even if that's all I'm doing, I'm recovering from major surgery.

Next month is February and that's an important month: it contains Valentine's Day of course, and then my first anniversary with Seb on the twentieth. After everything life has thrown at us, we're going to celebrate our anniversary in a few weeks' time, and that's something to be thankful for.

I'm healing up from my surgery: my mastectomy on my left side was a skin-sparing one so, although I've lost my nipple, there are fewer scars. No back muscle was removed, so I don't have to have physiotherapy to enable me to use my arm again like I had after my surgery on my right side.

Spitfire is the most beautiful and sweetest cat in the world. He likes to lie on his pink chair in the evening in front of the television. In the many hours of darkness we watch a lot of television – this is when we start getting into *Midsomer Murders,* having watched all the Agatha Christie ones, both *Poirot* and *Miss Marple*, as well as *Inspector Morse* and *Prime Suspect,* borrowed from my aunt and uncle.

Midsomer Murders is perfect post-operative viewing. Based on the books by Caroline Graham, Detective Chief Inspector Tom Barnaby, played by John Nettles, solves numerous murders that take place in the fictional English county of Midsomer.

Midsomer's main town, Causton, is based on Slough, apparently, but the little villages are just so pretty. There are usually three or four murders per episode. Sometimes the murders themselves are inventive and gruesome and the characters are a range of English eccentrics. I love *Midsomer Murders* so much and never tire of watching the antics of Barnaby and his sidekick.

Lying on the sofa, under my furry blanket, watching the murders, hospital seems far away. I just have to take my aromatase inhibitor pill every day, I tell myself, and go for my Zoladex injections every three months, and I can stay out of hospital and have a life. I still have to take my carbamazepine and duloxetine for my mental disorder of course, but at the moment my mood is up and life is good. I'm with the love of my life and we're happy. I'm enjoying Spin and becoming thinner and fitter, as well as making new friends in my class.

Considering ten months ago I was diagnosed with secondary breast cancer, it seems pretty amazing that here I am, doing so well. My oncologist hadn't known whether or not I'd respond to the Zoladex and letrozole and yet I'm apparently fit and healthy. I don't know what's going on in my lungs because I haven't had any scans for a while, but I certainly have reasons to be cheerful in the New Year.

"I love you, Fluffy Monster," I say to Spitfire, stroking the back of his head and down his back. "You're the best cat in the world." I knew I had to have this kitten so Seb would have a reason to visit me, and against all the odds my plan has worked. Seb is my boyfriend. Sometimes I can't quite believe this, but it's true. *Thank you G-d and well done me*, I think, stroking the most beautiful and fluffiest cat in the world and grateful for how lucky I am.

Chapter 13

"Don't forget, it's Valentine's Day soon," I say to Seb when we're chatting on the phone one evening. It's early February. Ginuary is over. Seb is in Exeter at university. I'm still at my parentals recuperating from my chest surgery.

"I won't forget, my lovely," Seb says. "I've got you something already. I'll stick it in the post."

"Oh, how exciting," I say. "Thank you, darling."

I'm up in Spitfire's bedroom which doubles as Mum's study. Mum has recently had the walls painted buttercup yellow and there are yellow blinds which are always left open so the Fluffy Monster doesn't get himself tangled up in them.

"So, when are you coming down?" I ask, looking in Mum's diary which lies on the desk, open to this week.

"Soon. This weekend I hope, depending on work," Seb says. "I've got a project to do about genetics in a frog pond – it's a computer simulation and …"

"OK, darling," I say. "Your work takes priority so …"

"I'll let you know when I can come down, my lovely," Seb says. "I've got to get on with some work now."

"Speak tomorrow, then," I say, feeling sad he has to go.

"Bye, my lovely," he says.

"Bye," I say, putting the phone down, feeling deflated, deprived of his mellifluous voice.

I miss Seb so much when he's not here. Leaving Spitfire's room I walk out into the hall. The marble floor is cold through my socks. The thing is, of course I want him to do well at university. This is his chance to make something of his life after the acting didn't work out and nor did the monastery. I must put my feelings to one side and concentrate on living my life here and let him do his work. *There's nothing to worry about*, I tell myself as I walk down the stairs, past Mum's orchid collection and into the kitchen. He hasn't met anyone else, I know this. *He wants to be with me*, I think, turning the tap on, filling the kettle to the two cup line. Standing by the kettle, I wait for it to boil. It's just: when I was at university, we partied all the time and still managed to complete our essays, whereas Seb has made one friend – just one – so I don't see why he can't get his work done in time to come down and see me at a weekend. *He must have more work for a science subject than I had for history*, I think.

Not that I'd be able to cope with a university course now, but my brain has sustained damage from years of mental illness and the treatments for it. His hasn't. He ought to be able to juggle the demands of a university course and a relationship.

The water boils. I fill my cup almost to the brim with milky coffee and then head out into the garden. Crossing the terrace, walking down the steps, I see Spitfire sharpening his claws on the wooden frame of the swinging chair.

"Hello, my Fluffy," I say, stroking his head.

Ignoring me, he makes to climb the sloping wooden pole but then seems to think better of it and returns to scratching. Furry, our previous cat, used to bound up the pole and stalk along the top, but Spitfire has short legs: Ragdolls are sturdy cats and not very agile. He decides to stay on the ground where he's safe.

Sitting on the swinging chair, holding my coffee, kicking the ground, I swing. From here I have a view over the grass towards the back of the house. Everything looks very wintery: the branches of the trees are bare, skeletons against the grey sky.

Mum comes out of the house, heads down the stairs towards me.

"I've got to go into the village, darling," she says. "Do you want to come?"

"OK," I say, draining my coffee. "I just need to get changed and …"

"Just put some of your gym leggings on and a sweater and a coat," Mum says, looking at my dressing gown, pyjamas and slippers. "Come on, I want to go in five minutes."

"OK," I say, getting up, heading back into the house.

In my bedroom I open the bottom drawer containing my gym clothes and take out my navy leggings with the rainbow tiger stripes down the side. It's cold so I change my knickers and socks and pull the leggings on as quickly as possible. I put on a black secret support top and then a black long-sleeved top over it.

"Come on, I want to go," I hear Mum saying outside my bedroom.

"I'm ready," I say, entering the bathroom, cleaning my teeth. "I just need my boots and …"

"They're in the hall," Mum says.

Running up the stairs in my socks, I find my black FitFlop boots in the hall and pull them on. I take my black coat from the coat rack and put on my grey eternity scarf, wrapping it twice round my neck.

In the car, I fiddle with my phone, turning it on, just in case a message arrives from Seb.

"Can we go to the Health Food shop?" I say, doing up my seatbelt.

"I have to get some milk and eggs and vegetables from Budgens," Mum says.

"I'll go to the Health Food shop and come and find you in Budgens then," I say, getting out of the car.

"There's a parcel for you," Dad says, the next day when I return from Spin. He hands me a padded envelope. Recognising Seb's writing on the front, I feel it: it feels soft and malleable. So, it's either an item of clothing or a soft toy.

"It's here," I text Seb. "Thank you, darling."

"You're not to open it till Valentine's Day," Seb's message says.

"I won't," I say. *I can try not to open it*, I think, *but I may not be able to stop myself.* If it's an animal in there he'll need to get out to breathe, after all. It's cruel to keep him cooped up in a padded envelope. I put it on my dressing table.

"Seb has sent a Valentine's Day present and made me promise not to open it. What shall I do?" I text my cousin Patrick's wife Julia. *She's experienced in the ways of men and the world, she'll know what to do*, I think.

"Open it, see what it is and then seal it up again, and pretend to Seb you haven't opened it," Julia messages back.

Opening the package, I pull out a fox soft toy. He's terracotta red with a white tummy and has some beads inside his bottom to weigh him down as he sits up. I love him, of course I do, but I can't shake a feeling of disappointment that, yet again, like the Christmas present of the dressing gown, this isn't a romantic gift. It's not jewellery, or underwear. *It's not what a boyfriend gives his girlfriend of a year for Valentine's Day*, I think, stroking my new fox. *Seb knows I like soft toys, though*, I think. And he is a top-of-the-range Jellycat one, a designer one no less. Putting my disappointment to one side, squashing it, I kiss my new fox on his face. I'm going to call him Freddy, I decide, after Freddy Fox, the actor. Also, Seb knows the Fox acting dynasty, so this is an apt name for my new fox. *I mustn't be disappointed*, I tell myself, stroking Freddy. *Seb is my boyfriend. For the first time in years I'm going to have a boyfriend on Valentine's Day and he's sent me a present. Everything is fine.*

It's February the twentieth, my anniversary with Seb. Approaching the restaurant where I'm meeting my cousins for lunch, I see him sitting on a bench near the bus stop and wave at him. He sees me and smiles, standing up, lifting his huge rucksack. He crosses the road, and we embrace.

"My darling, you're here," I say, kissing him. Seb is never on time, he's always late and yet here he is, on time, if not in fact early.

"I was at my brother's last night," he says, "and I got the bus, and I was early."

"I can't believe you're actually coming to a Cousins' Lunch," I say. "I'm so happy you're here."

"Me too," he says, kissing my forehead as we go to the restaurant.

We see my brother Carl sitting outside at the front of the restaurant, reading a book.

"Hello," I say.

"Hi," my brother says, putting his book away. "Hi Seb, how are you?"

"Very well," Seb says, taking a seat next to my brother.

A waiter comes out with some drinks menus, and we order gin and tonics and a beer for Carl.

"So, it's our first anniversary today," I say. "Mine and Seb's, so …"

"Happy anniversary," my brother says. Seb and I clink glasses and then we both clink our glasses against my brother's beer bottle.

"To us," I say, gazing into Seb's turquoise eyes. "Well done us." *I'm so happy he's here*, I think. *I'm so happy that at last he's come to a family event with me. I'm a normal person, going to a family lunch with my boyfriend.*

"To us," Seb says, putting his arm round me.

"We have an unusual relationship, but I think we make it work," I say, as we go into the restaurant to join the others. We can see some of them sitting at a long table already.

"We certainly do have an unusual relationship, my lovely," Seb says, smiling at me. Sitting down with Seb on one side of me, and Julia on the other, opposite my brother and Patrick, I pick up the menu and start to think about what I'm going to order.

Chapter 14

"I need something to help me through left-side radiotherapy," I say to Amber Rose, the owner of Destiny Rising, the New Age shop at the farm. I'm looking at the tray of rings that sit on the glass table in the middle of the shop. "How about this one?" I say, picking up a silver ring which is a dragon's head with a rainbow opal in the centre. His tail curls under him, round the finger. I love this ring, it's perfect.

"Wear it with the head looking out, away from your body, and he'll protect you," Amber Rose says, smiling at me. Her silver bangles jangle and as someone opens the door, the breeze blows through the dreamcatchers and wind chimes, which tinkle.

"OK, I'll take this," I say.

"That's thirty-eight pounds then," Amber Rose says. She is pretty: tanned, long blonde hair, looks about forty. Could be older: I'm no good at working out people's ages.

"Didn't you have radiotherapy a couple of years ago?" she asks, printing off the receipts, handing me mine.

"Yes, that was for my right side though," I say. "Now I have to have it for the other side and …"

"You want some smoky quartz," she says. "That's the cancer stone."

Turning round, I see all the little semi-precious stones in their trays. I choose a piece of smoky quartz and pay cash for it.

"Keep this with you all the time," she says.

"I'll keep it in my pouch for the moment," I say, putting it into my blue bum-bag which I wear most of the time. "Thank you."

"Enjoy your ring," she says, smiling as I leave the shop.

Opening the door, the dreamcatchers flutter, the wind chimes tinkle. Twisting my dragon ring, I feel prepared for the rigours of left-side radiotherapy.

"So, you need to hold your breath for thirty seconds, not letting it out at all," the radiologist says. I'm sitting on a chair in the radiotherapy room, not up on the machine. This is just a trial run to see if I can work the equipment. I have a mask over my face and a peg on my nose.

"Breathe in," the radiologist says. "And hold."

Breathing in, I want to start letting my breath out slowly, like when I'm swimming, but I mustn't. Holding my breath in, I hold it and hold it and then let it go.

"Twenty-two seconds," she says. "Not bad. But you have to be able to hold your breath for thirty seconds. Do you think you'll be able to do it or…"

"What happens if I can't?" I ask.

"Well, we had an older lady who couldn't," she says. "And that was OK. But it's much better if you can hold your breath. You can practise over the weekend, but you have to tell me now whether you're going to hold your breath or not, because how we set up the machine depends on that – we have to give you an extra layer of protection to wear and …"

"I'm going to do it," I say. "I'm going to hold my breath."

"Good girl, I'm pleased to hear it," she says. "It's much better for your heart if you can hold your breath as it holds your chest wall away from your heart, so it won't get damaged – your heart's just on your left side and …"

"I'm going to do it," I say. I'm a healthy thirty-seven-year-old. There's no reason why I can't hold my breath for thirty seconds. I'm determined to do it.

"Excellent. See you on Monday," she says, taking the mask away from me.

"See you on Monday," I say.

Over the weekend, I practise holding my breath. It's not easy to hold it without letting any out at all, not like underwater swimming where you gradually let your breath out until you need to take the next one. This is: breathe in sharply, hold for thirty seconds then breathe out sharply. It's difficult. And I will have to do it three times each session and repeat every day for three weeks. Radiotherapy has changed since last time I had it – now it's three weeks rather than five, and even higher doses. Because I had cancer in my skin last time, I have to have three times the normal dose. And left-side radiotherapy is demonstrably worse than right side, due to the breath-holding to keep the chest wall away from the heart.

"You need to take a breath until you can see you're in between the two lines, hold for thirty seconds and then release," the radiologist says.

I'm lying on the board with a bolster behind my lower back, wrists held in the supports, arms stretched out and held up, naked from the waist up. I'm wearing my new dragon ring and my bracelet and necklace from Seb. I'm sporting a mask and a pair of goggles with a screen, on which I can see two lines, and I have to breathe in and hold my breath between them and hold it without dropping below the lines for thirty seconds, then release.

Breathing in sharply, I go too far above the line, let a bit of breath out but too much comes out and I fall below the bottom line.

"Don't worry," the radiologist's voice says, from the other room. "Let your breathing return to normal then try again. We won't start the machine till you're ready."

Breathing in, I see my dot on the screen resting between the two lines. Holding my breath, I hear the machine whirring around me. Holding, holding, holding. I hold my breath. I see the straight line of my breath on the screen. The seconds pass with agonising slowness. Starting to feel dizzy, I keep holding my breath. That's fifteen seconds. Mustn't lose it now. Twenty seconds. It seems incredible how long a second can be. Twenty-five seconds. Somehow, the last five seconds pass and I've held my breath for thirty seconds.

"And release," the voice says. Letting my breath out, I see the line drop on the screen.

"Very good," the radiologist's voice says. "Now, when you're ready we're going to do it again."

I practise taking a deep breath in. The trick must be to get it just right and …

"Breathe normally," the radiologist says. "Let your breathing recover. We'll try again in a minute."

Breathing normally, I start to feel stressed about the fact that in a minute I'm going to have to hold my breath for thirty seconds. *It's OK*, I tell myself. *I can do this, I've just done it after all.*

"Breathe in and hold," the radiologist says.

Taking a big breath in, I see I've overshot the second line. I let out a bit of breath, but it's too much and falls below the first line.

"OK, breathe normally," the radiologist's voice says.

My breathing returns to normal.

"Breathe in," she says.

Breathing in sharply, I hit just between the two lines and hold, hold, hold. The machine whirrs into position. Five seconds pass, ten. The line of my breath on the screen is straight and lengthening. Time passes with agonising slowness. Desperate to let my breath out, I focus and hold it in. Fifteen seconds. *Just fifteen more seconds to go*, I think. *That's not long.* It is, in fact, long. Twenty seconds, twenty-five seconds. Feeling dizzy and exhausted I'm desperate to breathe. *Just five more seconds to go.*

"And release," the radiologist's voice says. I start to breathe again.

"Very good," she says. "Now, we're just going to put the bolus on and then we'll do all that again."

Another radiologist comes in, carrying the bolus. It is a sheet of gel-like plastic, and its job is to direct the radiation further down into the skin. She places it onto my chest and fixes it in place with bits of tape. The bolus is cold, heavy and uncomfortable. *Must enjoy breathing*, I think. The radiologist leaves the room and I'm alone again in my mask, with the machine. Looking into my goggles, I see the lines that I have to hold my breath between.

"Breathe in and hold," the radiologist says.

Taking a big breath in, I hold it between the two lines. Holding my breath, I hear the machine whirr round. Five seconds. Focusing on the line creeping across the screen, holding my breath, that's ten seconds. It's dark in the room, on my own. *This is the last time*, I think. *Just a few more seconds and then I can go home.* Fifteen seconds. *Can't wait for this to be over.* Twenty seconds. Starting to feel dizzy but have to keep holding my breath. Twenty-five seconds. *Just five more seconds to go and then it's over.*

"That's it," the radiologist's voice says. "Release and breathe normally. Well done, that's all for today."

Letting my breath go, I'm so happy to be able to breathe again. *That was tough*, I think. *And I'm going to have to do it all again tomorrow.*

The lights come on.

"Well done," the radiologist says, coming into the room to take the bolus off me, lowering the part of the machine that I'm lying on so I can get down. "You can get dressed now."

Taking my wrists out of the supports, I sit up, swinging my legs over to one side of the bed. Climbing down, crossing the room in my socks, I sit on the chair to put my shoes on and then pull my secret support vest top over my head and then my long-sleeved top.

"Bye," I say to the radiologists as I walk past the room where they're sitting. Mum is in the waiting room.

"How was it?" she asks.

"It was hard work," I say. "But I did it."

"Well done, darling," she says, putting her arm round me. "Let's go home."

"So, I have to breathe in," I say to Seb on the phone that evening. "And then hold my breath for thirty seconds, without letting it out at all. And I have to do it three times and …"

"Can you meditate whilst you're holding your breath?" Seb says.

"Not really," I say, stroking the Fluffy Monster who's lying on my parents' bed next to me. "I have to look at a screen so I can't really meditate or …"

"I wish I could come down this weekend, my lovely," Seb says. "But I've got too much work, I can't possibly drive down and …"

"Don't worry, darling." I say, although I wish he could visit, I really do. The problem is that it's a six-hour drive, at least, and he needs to get on with his work.

"I've got something I have to get in for Monday," Seb says. "But the puppy is coming soon and then I'll take you to see him, I promise."

"Oh, I can't wait to see him," I say. "When is he coming?"

"I think they're going to Wales to pick him up this weekend," Seb says. Seb's mum and stepdad are getting a new puppy and soon, very soon, I'll be able to meet him. I'm so excited. It's good to have something to look forward to.

"I have to go my lovely," Seb says. "I need to have some supper and get on with my work and …"

"Speak tomorrow, darling." I say, feeling sad he has to go already and so disappointed that I won't see him this weekend. *Ah well*, I think, *I must practise my breathing.*

"Miaow," Spitfire says, stretching.

"Would you like some supper, darling?" I ask.

Jumping off the bed, he stalks across the floor, turning his head to make sure I'm following him. Crossing the hall, padding across the marble floor, he enters his room and sits next to his bowl, looking up at me.

"OK, my Fluffy," I say, taking the container of dried food down from the bookshelf, and pouring it into his bowl.

Lowering his face, he starts crunching through his dried food. Tiptoeing out of the room, I leave him to eat his supper.

Chapter 15

"Hold still," Mum says. I'm lying on my bed and she's placing a gauze pad over the severe burn on my left side and fixing it to the undamaged skin around it with pink Micropore tape. The hospital gave me gel pads to cool the burnt skin but that hasn't really worked, the skin is peeling off anyway, so here we are, bandaging it.

"Ouch," I say. "That hurts."

"Nearly done, darling," Mum says, taping around the edges of the gauze pad with the tape, pressing it down whilst attempting not to hurt me. She hurts me a lot. The horrors of breath-holding and the three weeks of left-side radiotherapy are now over, just the severe burns to deal with now.

It's March and I haven't seen Seb for weeks. *I miss him*, I think as I put my top on and flinch from the pain.

"Hello, my lovely," Seb says when he calls. "I've spoken to my mum and we can visit the puppy this weekend and …"

"Oh that's wonderful," I say, feeling excited. "I can't wait to meet him. How's he settling in?"

"Well, he's not taking very well to sleeping in the kitchen," Seb says. "So he's been sleeping in bed with my mum and my stepdad, but other than that he's settling in well I think."

"I can't wait to see him and cuddle him," I say. "I'm so excited. Thank you so much for arranging it, darling. How's your work going?"

"I'm getting on with it," Seb says, not sounding too convinced. "I'd better get back to it now, in fact, so …"

"OK, my darling," I say. "See you at the weekend."

"Goodbye, my lovely," Seb says. "Call you tomorrow."

"My lovely, please don't be upset but I'm not going to be able to come down this weekend," Seb says when he calls the next day.

"Oh, that's such a shame," I say, feeling devastated. "How come?"

"Well, I got my piece of work back, the one about genetics in the frog pond," he says, sounding upset. "Unfortunately, I got a terrible mark in it, I obviously didn't understand what I was meant to be doing or … well, I need to stay here really and get on with my work and …"

"OK, darling," I say. "Obviously your work is the most important thing so …"

"I'm so terribly sorry," he says. "I really wanted to take you to see the puppy this weekend and …"

"Don't worry, my darling," I say, trying to keep the disappointment out of my voice. "We'll see the puppy soon or …"

"Thank you for being so understanding," Seb says. "I'll call you tomorrow."

"Bye, my darling," I say, putting the phone down.

Throwing myself down on my parental bed – the phone doesn't work in my area of the house – I burst into tears. I haven't seen Seb for weeks, almost a month. I've been so much looking forward to seeing him and to meeting the puppy this weekend. His work is important, of course it is, but I've just finished radiotherapy and I feel weak and exhausted and I just want to see my boyfriend. *I just don't understand why everything always conspires against us*, I think, as I sob into my 'mum's pillow. *I don't ask for much from life, I just want to see my boyfriend sometimes. I never complain about all the horrible treatments or about my mental disorder or anything. The only thing I want is to see my Seb, and yet again I can't.*

"Supper time," Mum says, putting her head round the door. "What's the matter, darling?" Mum looks concerned.

"Don't worry," I say, sitting up, blowing my nose. "Let's go and have some supper."

"You have to tell me what's wrong," Mum says, as we sit down at the table. "I can't look after you properly if you don't tell me what's going on or …"

"Seb got a bad mark in a piece of work," I say, gulping back tears. "And so he has to stay in Exeter this weekend and so we're not going to meet the puppy and …" Tears are tumbling down my cheeks and falling into my open mouth. I'm gasping for air because I'm crying so much.

"Oh, I'm sorry, darling," Mum says. "I know how much you were looking forward to it so …"

"It's OK," I say. "I'll see him soon and …"

"Come on, eat your supper," Mum says.

Looking at my plate, I see a scrambled egg with cheddar and mushrooms sitting on two slices of toast, broccoli and cauliflower. Crying has given me a headache and I don't feel hungry, but I know Mum will be cross with me if I don't eat my supper so I cut off a small piece of scrambled egg on toast and I wash it down with some wine. After a couple of glasses of Rioja I feel better and am able to eat the rest of my supper.

At least it's March now, we're over the bit of the year I really hate – January and February, I think. *Soon I will see Seb*. The rugby is on and Seb loves rugby so I watch it, trying to understand it. It's easy enough to work out what's going on when the ball is in play and you can see it, but I don't understand what's happening in the scrums and rucks without Seb to explain it to me. Still, I watch it so I can talk to him about it when he calls. It is good to have a new sport to learn about.

"I'm definitely coming to see you at the end of term, my lovely," Seb says when he calls. "Term finishes on the 27th and we'll go out for some drinks and then I'll come up the next day and …"

"Excellent," I say. "I look forward to seeing you then and …"

"Then we'll go and see the puppy," Seb says.

"Have all your siblings seen him?" I ask.

"'Fraid so, my lovely," Seb says. "We're the last ones to meet him."

"Well, it's not long now," I say. "Soon it will be the end of term and we can meet him." *And see each other*, I think.

"Bunny likes small dogs," Seb's brother says to me. We're sitting on the sofa with Doodle in between us. Buster – the Labrador – rests his head against my knee. Stroking him, I look at Edward. He's darker, shorter and squatter than Seb but in fact I've got far more in common with *him* – he read English at Magdalen College, Oxford. His wife, Bunny, is a lawyer. So is Edward. I like him a lot, but this is the first time I've met Bunny. Seb has told me again and again about how he doesn't get on with her so I'm surprised to find her warm, funny and easy to talk to.

"I'm the opposite," I say. "I'm a gigantophile. I like really big dogs."

"Oh, me too," Edward says. "Me too. But Bunny just likes them when they're small so this is our second visit already."

"I wouldn't have thought of getting a present for the puppy," Bunny says. "That's so sweet of you."

"Of course I got him a present," I say, watching the puppy destroy the please-be-gentle-with-this-toy one. He is three-quarters golden Labrador and one-quarter poodle. He is adorable.

"That toy's not going to last long," Seb says, coming in from the garden. He's probably been helping his mum with something – he's always helping his mum move chairs and so on. There's a wedding happening tomorrow at the barn next door to the house where Seb's mum and stepdad hold weddings, so we all have to get out of the way by tomorrow morning.

"There's another toy," I say. "One that's a bit tougher I think."

"Let's give him that one then," Seb says, taking it out of the packet. But the puppy has fallen asleep now and he is lying on his back with his round pink tummy exposed, snoring.

"Yes, Buster," Seb says, sitting next to me. "I love you." Stroking the Labrador's grizzled head, he bends to kiss him. "We will always have our relationship. I will always play Frisbee with you. Don't worry."

Buster is not pleased about the new puppy and sticks close to us, pawing us for strokes and cuddles.

"Now, you mustn't ignore my other dogs," Seb said in the car on the journey.

"I can't believe you'd think I would do that," I said. "If anything, I'll give Buster and Doodle extra attention because I'm so sensitive to the fact that there's a new puppy and they must be feeling neglected."

"Good," Seb said. "Glad to hear it. You are sweet, my lovely."

I am sweet, I think now, sitting next to Seb on the sofa, with Doodle between us and Buster resting against Seb's legs. *I am sweet and Seb is lucky to have me.* I wonder whether he realises this or whether he thinks any girlfriend would put up with everything I put up with: the long absences; his timekeeping; his banging on about wanting to be a celibate monk. I know I'm lucky to have him but sometimes I wonder whether or not he knows he's lucky to have me: my unwavering devotion; my willingness to walk through fire for him; the fact I've waited for eleven years.

"Darling," I say, quietly. "Is it OK if I go up and have a sleep now?"

"I'll come with you," Seb says, standing up. "OK, Ed, Bunny, we're going up to have a sleep. See you at supper."

"See you later," Ed and Bunny chorus.

Mounting the stairs, we arrive at the top, past the not-very-good painting of the horse that Seb or one of his siblings painted – or that's what I presume, I've never asked where the painting

came from, I realise. We're in a different room from last time –
Seb's old bedroom, which is yellow. There are some books about
animals on the bookshelves and a large long-haired tortoiseshell
cat on the bed.

"Hello Fatby," I say, reaching out a hand to stroke her. She's
Spitfire's half-sister, from a previous litter of Kitty's. She is the biggest
of all the cats.

Changing into a secret support top and some pants, I get into
bed. Seb takes his trousers off and climbs in next to me. The cat
jumps off the bed and stalks out of the room.

Seb falls asleep almost immediately. I watch him, his long lashes
grazing his tanned cheeks as he sleeps, his arm thrown around me.
This is what it's all for, I think, gazing at him, completely mine in his
sleep. *This is what it's all for: all the waiting, all the missing him – here
we are together at last*. And as I watch him sleep and feel his strong
arm around me, I begin to relax. *Everything is OK*, I think. *We're
together, it's the Easter holidays and then it's going to be summer. We're
going to be able to spend some time together – go to the zoo, maybe go
on holiday together. We've been separated but now we're together and
everything is going to be wonderful like it was last summer. I love him so
much, my darling, darling boyfriend.*

Why I Drink

- I drink to dull my inner pain that breast cancer and bipolar 1
  have taken away my chances of a career and husband.
- I drink with Seb to paper over the cracks in our relationship.
- To allow me to socialise and to be on good form.
- To be funny and forget the void at my core.
- To anaesthetise myself against the reality that life is cruel, and I
  have been dealt a tough hand.

- To feel "the click" that Brick talks about in *Cat on a Hot Tin Roof*, where I'm drunk enough to cope with the vicissitudes of life.
- When I'm bored watching television because I shun my friends who don't like to watch me drink at lunchtime.
- To fall asleep.
- After Seb split up with me and I stop taking carbamazepine, to suppress the wren of anxiety. Alcohol withdrawal causes anxiety which I must avoid at all costs.
- I start twitching about 11.30am due to alcohol withdrawal so have my first gin and tonic then, or even kosher wine when that's all they have at the Israeli beach bar.
- To fill the huge space left when Seb is gone for good.
- To deal with my disfigured body and lack of hair from cancer treatment.
- To seize the day: I'm not dead yet. May as well be in a drunken stupor.
- Habitually: with food as my parents drink – less than me – at dinner time.
- To quiet the panther's negative comments.
- To calm my racing thoughts when hypomanic.
- I love the ritual of cocktail hour: making my cocktail and then drinking it slowly.
- To give a structure to my aimless life: first drink at eleven thirty; drinks with lunch; then afternoon drunken sleep; then coffee; then cocktail at six o'clock – cocktail hour – then wine with and after dinner.

PART TWO

Chapter 16

APRIL 2016

"Here you go," I say, mixing up the dry and wet food, standing against the kitchen counter. Behind me there's an enormous black dog with gold forelegs, gold eyebrows, gold around his muzzle, a gold throat and a long, silky black tail. His glossy ears hang down, and his coat shines. *He's the most beautiful creature in the world*, I think, as he lies there waiting for his breakfast. As I place it on the floor, he doesn't move. He's a well-trained person: he has to be – he's the size of a Shetland pony.

"Wait," I say, and he stays. "Now," I say, and he approaches the bowl and starts to chomp through his breakfast.

Putting the dirty fork in the sink, I go upstairs. It's 7.15 a.m. Mustn't wake up Mary. I'm awake, of course, because my mood is up. We're dog-sitting for Cato the Hovawart whilst his owners are in South Africa on a wildlife reserve.

At the top of the landing, I pass the closed door to Mary's room and open the one to the master bedroom where I'm staying. Sitting on the bed, I take my zebra bag containing my meds out of my suitcase and count out my duloxetine and fexofenadine, sodium docusate and ibuprofen. I have a headache. I have a constant headache. That's apparently down to the letrozole but it could also be caffeine withdrawal. Sipping my coffee, I think about the day ahead.

Soon Mary will wake up and then it will be an hour since Cato's breakfast and we can walk him. He needs to digest his breakfast as big dogs are prone to stomach torsion: that's where their stomach twists, and it can be fatal. So, he has to digest his breakfast before we walk him, just to be safe.

It's 8.03 a.m. *OK, let's see if Mary is up*, I think. Knocking on the door, I hear her say "Yes?"

Opening the door, I walk into the room and sit on the bed.

"Good morning, darling," I say. "I've given Cato his breakfast and …"

"Oh good," Mary says, rubbing her eyes. "I slept really well. How did you sleep?"

"I slept OK," I say. "I'm going to go and have some breakfast and …"

"See you downstairs in a bit," Mary says.

We're walking across the fields. I'm wearing my black FitFlop boots – it's a bit muddy but not impossible to walk. The sun is shining.

"How are you feeling?" Mary asks. I'm holding the lead and although Cato is quite strong I think I'm keeping up with him without allowing him to pull me along too fast.

"Yeah, OK," I say. "Quite cheerful – I mean my mood is OK – just tired and …"

"Well, we've just got to do a five mile walk," she says.

"Oh, that sounds nice," I say but the thought of walking for five miles – it sounds far too long. I don't mind a bit of a trek, but five whole miles seems beyond me.

There is an enormous thing in my mind – the elephant in the room – that I mustn't think about.

We trudge through the mud.

"This seems like such a long walk," I say, trying not to complain but …

111

"You know what they say," Mary says. "Country miles are longer."

I can't wait to sit down, I think. *It will be so nice when this walk is over.*

Back at the house, we open the gate, open the back door. Sitting down at the big wooden kitchen table, I watch Mary put the kettle on. Cato comes in and lies at my feet.

"Seb told me he'd stay with me 'til the end," I say. "But he didn't and …"

"That was naughty of him, saying that," Mary says, bringing my coffee over, sitting down at the table with me.

"I don't know how I'm going to live without him," I say, feeling the tears starting to come. I've been crying myself to sleep for a couple of hours every night since Seb split up with me a week ago, and I've come to Suffolk to help Mary house-and-dog-sit for a bit of a break, but I just feel so broken.

"You will," Mary says, putting her arm round me. "You will just gradually start to feel better – time will heal."

"He made it all seem OK – my illnesses, the horrible treatments and now … well now there's just my chronic mental disorder and my chronic terminal illness."

"There are things you enjoy doing which are nothing to do with him," Mary says. "Spin, going to the gym, being with Spitfire, being with dogs …"

"I just don't understand why he didn't think our relationship was worth saving," I say, reaching down to stroke Cato's head. I must not get down on the floor with him as then he'll get on top of me and I won't be able to get up. I remember this from my last visit here two summers ago. That summer: when Seb was away in the monastery in Thailand, but we were happy. The tears roll down my cheeks.

"It's going to get better than this," Mary says, putting her arm round me. "Why don't we find something to watch later?"

Walking through to the television room, Cato follows us, waving his huge brush of a tail.

"Oh look, here's *Vinyl*," Mary says. This is the series that I asked Cato's owners to record. Produced by Mick Jagger and starring his son, it's set in the New York record industry in the 1970s and I've heard excellent things about it. I'm looking forward to watching it. "They've already recorded a few episodes of it."

"Oh, good," I say. "We should go and get some food."

"OK, let's walk to Tesco," Mary says.

The house is on the Tesco estate – the shop is just a few minutes' walk away. Going back upstairs, I find my gold Puma trainers and pull them on. "Ready when you are," I say.

"We need wine," I say, picking up two bottles of Rioja. We have a basket full of spinach, eggs, feta and other groceries.

Mary looks at me. "Are you sure? I mean, surely one bottle of wine will be enough and ... I don't think you ought to be drinking so much. I know you're upset about Seb but it's not going to help and ..."

"If we don't finish two bottles that's fine," I say. "I'd just like to get both bottles just in case we finish one and ..."

"Well, we're not going to," Mary says, putting a bottle back on the shelf. "I've decided we're just getting one bottle, which is quite enough wine for two of us for one day so ..."

"Fine," I say, but I start to feel anxious. I'm going to want a glass of wine with lunch and then at least two or three with supper and I'm already starting to twitch because I haven't had a drink yet today and it's 11.30 a.m.

Back at the house, Mary makes lunch. Sitting at the kitchen table, I stroke the top of Cato's enormous, soft head. I'm thinking about Seb. I'm thinking about what Seb is doing right now. I wonder if he's still at his brother's, at his 'mum's or back in Exeter. After speaking every day for thirteen months, not hearing from him is tough. *I am addicted to him*, I think, and the tears roll down my cheeks.

The delicious smell of baked omelette wafts over to me from the oven.

"Nearly ready," Mary says.

Walking over to where I can see the bottle of Rioja sitting by the sink, I pick it up and open it with the corkscrew. *Soon, in a few moments, I will have a glass of wine and I will begin to feel better.* Pouring a glass, I sniff it and the strong bouquet hits me. Feeling calmer, I sit down and wait for my lunch.

"This is lovely," I say to Mary as I taste the baked leek, feta and pepper omelette.

"Good, I'm glad you like it," she says. "I have to feed Diego after lunch, do you want to come with or …"

"I'll stay here and have a sleep," I say. Diego is a Ragamuffin cat – he is silver and looks like Spitfire but slimmer and smaller "a fluffy tail with a cat attached" as Mary says. She calls him "the snow leopard".

Mary leaves after lunch to feed Diego. Opening the freezer, I see a bottle of vodka. Pouring a couple of inches into a glass, I top it up with tonic and take it up to my room. Draining the glass, I take off my leggings and climb into bed. Closing my eyes, I see Seb splitting up with me at my flat and start crying and continue for about forty minutes until I pass out.

Waking up with a start and a headache, pulling on my pyjama trousers, I creep downstairs. Mary isn't back yet so I pour myself another vodka and Slimline tonic and also put some oats into a coffee cup. Squeezing some honey onto them, I make a cup of coffee too. Taking my two drinks and my snack back upstairs, I settle back into bed to write my blog.

Hearing the front door open, I knock back my vodka – I don't even like it but needs must – and clean my teeth so Mary can't smell it on my breath, at least I hope she won't be able to. Picking up my cup of coffee, I head downstairs.

"How was the snow leopard?" I ask. Mary is sitting in the living room. Cato lies on the floor in front of her sofa. He's not allowed on the furniture.

"He was alright," Mary says, stroking her hair behind her ear. "He was sad when I had to go, he doesn't like being on his own."

"I'll come with you tomorrow," I say, sipping my coffee, feeling really tired.

We're all in the living room after supper, watching *Vinyl*. It's brilliant: gripping, funny, evoking the place and period – the New York record industry in the seventies – with flair and panache and a lot of drugs. James Jagger as the young musician and Juno Temple as the A & R girl are both great, but it's Bobby Cannavale as the hero who delivers the stand-out performance.

As we watch the programme, I drink.

"I just went to fill my glass up and the wine was almost finished," Mary says, looking concerned.

I knew we should've got two bottles.

"Oh, have I had that much, I'm sorry, I didn't realise," I say, even though of course I realise – I'm not stupid. "It's good, isn't it, *Vinyl*? I'm really enjoying it, are you?"

"Yes, it's wonderful," Mary says, sounding excited. "Good choice – I love it."

Suddenly I'm tired, I'm so tired, I just want to go to bed.

"I'm going to bed," I say. "See you in the morning."

"Sleep well," Mary says, smiling at me.

"Goodnight, darling boy," I say, stroking Cato's head. He wags his huge feathery tail. He's so gorgeous – he's the most beautiful dog I've ever seen.

Climbing the stairs, I wobble. I'm cutting down my antidepressant and mood stabiliser in preparation for changing to a different antidepressant and an antipsychotic – maybe it's that making me not feel well. Or maybe I've just had too much to drink. Or maybe I'm coming down with something. Washing my evening meds down with a glass of water, I climb into bed and cry about Seb for an hour or so. I miss him so much. We always used to speak every evening. Then I pass out into a dreamless sleep.

Chapter 17

Once upon a midnight dreary
Whilst you wandered, weak and weary
Here's the raven, here he comes
He uses tools
He'd use his thumbs
If thumb's'd been granted
To him. He sits on your porch
The light is dim
From his perch above your door
Quoth the raven **Nevermore**
An old-time harbinger of news
Your psychic gifts today must use
You feed him: Apollo's messenger of bad news
You scratch his head
What's wrong you said
The raven answers **Nevermore**
What other words, black sprite
You say
The raven stays at break of day
The golden chariot of the sun
Phaeton steals the chariot once
From his dad Helios, the dunce
He drives our sun across the sky

Helios sits on diamond-studded throne
Steer the sun chariot through a middle course
Helios tells his boy, and then
Do not go too high or low
My fiery horses take no shit
I know you think now that you're it
But son of mortal that you be
Best leave my chariot to me.
Phaeton shakes his angry head
I won't, Dad, just won't end up dead.
Sun chariot blazes a gash in the sky
Our Milky Way now
Zeus, enraged, strikes Phaeton with thunderbolt
And then, Phaeton in Eridanus river falls
Heilandes transformed to poplar trees
To guard there their brother for all time
It's easy to maintain this rhyme.
But how's the raven on your door,
Quoth he again **Nevermore.**
He uses a stick as a tool
To fish bugs out of the wall.
And the silken sad uncertain rustling of each purple curtain
Thrills you, fills you with fantastic terrors never felt before.
And the raven stays nearby, you
Are you about to die, you wonder
Wonder this for evermore.
Is there, is there balm in Gilead
Is there, will there be respite
From this never-ending night
That the raven brings as he sits
Upon your chamber door

Quoth the raven ***Nevermore.***
What is it you forget now
You say. Why does night follow day
Why does Phaeton die
As he careers across the sky
Why is Zeus so cross
Why is there so much loss
Why are we tempest-tossed today
Why, does it always end this way.
The raven cleans his plumage dark,
The raven grasps above your door:
Quoth the raven ***Nevermore.***
Lenore is dead and with her love
Is your death coming now, for sure
It is. And some days hence,
The raven perches on your fence,
He watches you with demon eyes,
Nowhere else doth he fly.
He watches you, he doesn't go,
The sun sets now, here comes the snow.
The raven guards your property,
Now who are you and who is she
The raven stays, Hope vanishes
That you'll separate your life from his.
He is clever, he is kind
He controls now all your mind.
He is huge, with you he sits
Your self fragments, dissolves in bits.
No freedom now and no Lenore,
The raven sits there at your door.
He forages for woodlice, here

He drains the water,
Drains your tears,
He grooms his plumage every night,
Your heart is here, your soul takes flight.
Phaeton in chariot he roars,
Quoth the raven ***Nevermore.***

No more love knocks at your chamber door.

Chapter 18

APRIL 2016

"Did you drink this whole bottle of vodka?" Mary asks, picking up a bottle, showing it to me.

"No, I just had a couple of … I mean, I just had one or two drinks," I say, looking at her.

"This bottle was full at the beginning of the week," she says, not looking at me.

"Was it? I hadn't noticed," I say, looking out of the window at where the gigantic pooch is wandering in the garden outside, sniffing a bush.

"At the beginning of the week, this bottle was full," she says, sounding irritated. "And we've been drinking a bottle of wine a day, I mean you have. You've drunk a bottle of wine a day every day and a whole bottle of vodka in a week – I think you've got a problem."

"No, I haven't," I say, not looking at her.

"Look, this isn't going to wash with me," Mary says. "My mum was an alcoholic for years remember. This denial, this … do you want me to speak to your mum or …"

"No," I say, staring out of the kitchen window into the garden where the most beautiful dog in the world is now lying down, cleaning himself, licking his haunch with his long pink tongue. He has to keep that coat in perfect condition.

"I mean, I know you're under a lot of pressure now," she says. "After the split with Seb and … well, maybe you need someone to talk to and … I don't know – this denial and …"

"I'm sorry," I say, but I don't feel anything. I need to be drinking this amount to keep going at the moment and I don't see any point in discussing it. And maybe I should feel bad for worrying Mary when I know her mum used to be an alcoholic and it caused problems in her childhood but all I can think is *I can't deal with this, I need a drink.*

"I've had a text from Greg to say can we please replace the vodka," Mary says, looking at me, looking cross. "I'm sorry about my toxic negativity, I know I should be trying to be understanding and maybe even sympathetic, but I just find this so difficult so …"

"I'm sorry," I say. "Let's go – um where should we go to …"

"The vodka's probably from Tesco," Mary says. "That's where they get everything – since it's just round the corner."

"OK," I say. "Tesco."

"Come in, good boy," Mary says to the pooch, and he comes in, wagging his huge brush of a tail, walks past us and settles down in his bed in the hall, gnawing on his bone. We go out through the back door and walk in the direction of Tesco.

At Tesco we walk towards the drinks aisle and I find the correct vodka bottle and I'm so relieved that they've got it and I know I ought to be feeling so bad about how much I've been drinking and about drinking their vodka but I just put it to one side because I have to get on with the here and now which is getting through each day without Seb. The days stretch ahead of me "Like a Motorway" – all grey and long – that's Saint Etienne but it's all clichés now anyway. Seb is gone and I'm not really alive – just existing. Half of me has been ripped away – I've lost a limb.

On the train on the way home I buy two double gin and Slimline tonics and sit there in my seat, watching the flat East

Anglian landscape roll by. Egrets stand by a pond: a pair of ballerinas in white, motionless. *This should be rock bottom*, I think. I lost Seb because of my drinking or partly because of it and now I've really upset my best friend and this should be a wake-up call. This should be an epiphany that I have to change my life. This should be rock bottom: I've lost Seb and I've really upset my best friend who loves me – alcohol is ruining my relationships.

Ah well, I think, sipping my gin and tonic, thinking how good it tastes. *Life can wait – there's drinking to do.* Eating my cheese and pickle sandwich, I read my book, Ben Fogle's *Labrador: The Story of the World's Favourite Dog*, and suddenly I'm in Newfoundland, Canada with the fishermen and a tough all-purpose gun dog and retriever as he is transformed into the World's Favourite Pet.

Back at the parental home, I settle into a routine: Spin in the morning, first gin and Slimline tonic at 11.30 a.m., lunch, body scan meditation, sleep, wake up, walk, supper and more drinks.

"It's almost six o'clock," I say to Mum. We're in the kitchen, Mum is making supper and I'm standing next to her, waiting to be allowed my first glass of wine this evening. It's all I can think about at the moment: alcohol and the loss of Seb which has burnt a huge hole right through me. I wonder if Mum can see through into my chest where my heart is broken and bleeding. *It seems more than pointless to have put myself through the horrors of left-side radiotherapy to protect my heart when Seb has just broken it anyway*, I think.

"It's six o'clock now," I say.

"OK, darling, you can have a glass of wine. I'll have one too," Mum says, chopping up some cucumber to put in the salad.

Taking a bottle of wine out of the fridge, it's Torres Viña Sol, I pour out two glasses and put a piece of ice in each one.

"Here you go," I say to Mum, handing her a glass.

"Cheers," Mum says, smiling at me as we clink glasses.

The first sip of wine tastes so good.

"Where's my Fluffy?" I ask Mum.

"Sitting down on his black-and-white sofa," Mum says. "Why don't you take some olives and join him. I'll be with you in a minute and …"

"OK," I say, opening the drawer next to the fridge, taking out a small tin of olives stuffed with garlic and pouring the olives into the olive dish which has a special compartment for the stones. Carrying my glass of wine and the bowl of olives, I walk down the stairs to the living room and place them on the glass table.

Spitfire is stretched out on his black and white sofa: face pressed into the back of the sofa, long back legs and tail dangling over the end. He wakes up at my approach and turns over, hauling his back end up, starting to lick his haunches.

"Hello Fluffy Monster," I say, stroking him along the top of his head and down his back, where he likes to be stroked. He doesn't ignore me but doesn't bite me either, he accepts my attention as a deserved tribute to his wonderfulness.

Looking at my beautiful cat, feeling his softness, I feel so lucky to have him in my life. *It will be fine*, I think, sitting on the grey sofa next to him. *I'll cut down my drinking, I'll be well enough to return to work soon, I'll get over Seb, I'll just somehow pull my life back together. I've cut down my drinking before, I'll be able to do it again.* Putting an olive in my mouth, I look at the Fluffy Monster and he stares back at me with yellow eyes.

"I'm going to stop drinking so much," I tell him as I sip my wine. "Not today, but soon. I'm going to start drinking like a normal person. Who knows, I may well even start taking some days off from drinking like people do these days. It's not impossible."

Spitfire looks at me, yellow eyes wide. I wish I could know what he was thinking.

"It's just a tough time at the moment," I say, realising I've almost finished my glass of wine. "Seb's just split up with me and I'm not well enough to get back to work and …" I break off. Mum's in her bathroom. Running up the stairs to the kitchen, opening the fridge, I refill my glass of wine. Returning to the lounge, I sit back down on the grey sofa and sip my wine, so it looks as if I'm halfway down my first glass. Phew.

"It's our secret," I whisper to Spitfire. "Don't tell your grandma." I know this isn't good. I know this isn't what I want to be doing and yet I can't see a way to stop it. *At least the panther's not here*, I think. At least for the moment my mood is still holding and hasn't yet crashed. *I must be grateful for small mercies*, I tell myself, stroking Spitfire's soft, orange fur.

Chapter 19

Waking up, I realise the panther is lying on top of me.

"You're back," I say, although of course I don't need to for here he is – a huge dead weight pressing down on me.

"Did you miss me?" he asks, licking my ear, rasping it with his rough tongue.

"No, I didn't," I say. "In fact, I'd prefer it if you just return right now to wherever you've come from and …"

"No such luck, I'm afraid," he says. "You're stuck with me now."

So, here we are. The panther is back. I've had just four months without him. Pushing him away, sitting up in bed, I think *I want to die, I want to die, I want to die* over and over and over. There doesn't seem any point in trying to do anything, so I sit up in bed, waiting for Mum.

Hearing the tap, tap, tap of Mum's heels down the steps, I wait. She knocks on the door.

"Come in," I say.

"Good morning, darling," Mum says. "I brought someone to see you." Her arms are full of an enormous orange Fluffy Monster.

"What's that?" I ask, stroking his head.

"It's a wild lion," Mum says. "He just came into the house. He's very friendly." She deposits him on my bed. The panther regards him with pity, amber eyes wide, but Spitfire ignores the bigger cat and sits in the middle of my bed, grooming himself. He sticks out a long fluffy back leg and licks it clean.

"The panther's here," I say to Mum.

Mum sits on the edge of my bed: it's getting a bit crowded in here. "That's rotten luck, I'm sorry, darling," she says, stroking my hair. "How long …"

"Well, my mood was just up for four months," I say. "And now the panther's here and …"

"Well,, you'd better put your antidepressant dose up," Mum.

"Not that that has ever worked, no matter how many times we've tried it," I say.

"Well, that's the first thing to do," Mum says, in a decisive tone. "I'll bring you your porridge and coffee and then I'll take you to Spin. Maybe that will take your mind off it."

"Thank you," I say.

Mum leaves the room and Spitfire trots after her, thick fur pantaloons wobbling as he runs, huge brush of a tail held up behind him and waving in the air.

Eating my porridge, drinking my coffee, I think about Spin. Now the panther is here I dread even this, my favourite occupation. The music will seem too loud, my speed and strength will be affected and I will avoid talking to anyone. Breakfast finished, I take off my sleepwear and pull on knickers, sports bra, padded cycling shorts, vest top, leopard print leggings. Picking up my pouch, I fasten it round my waist. Slipping my feet into my white FitFlop moon boots, I pick up my powder-blue long-sleeved top from my chair and put it on. Going into the bathroom, I clean my teeth and wipe my face with a facial wipe.

Climbing the stairs to the kitchen, I open the drawer where my pills live and count out one fexofenadine, my allergy pill; two venlafaxine, my antidepressant; and two sodium docusate, the pills I've been taking since chemotherapy to stop the terrible constipation I suffer from, so severe my bum bleeds.

The panther sits outside the kitchen waiting for me. When I've taken my pills, I look around the house for Mum. She's already up in the hall, waiting for me. She's dressed in her tennis clothes: a pair of powder-pink shorts, white trainers, a white t-shirt and a pale pink zip-up fleece.

"Let's get going then," Mum says . The panther bounds ahead of me and as Mum opens the car door he jumps in and spreads out across the back seat. Mum puts her tennis bag in the boot. I sit in the front seat, looking at all the new green shoots on the new trees. It's spring – it's my favourite time of year. *I should be cheerful*, I think. But the weight of the world presses down on me.

"Talk to me, darling," Mum says, as she drives down the road. "Stop staring into space."

But I can't speak – I have such a deep sense of foreboding. And the wren of anxiety – we will meet her later – flaps down my throat into my stomach. I just stare out of the window at the trees as we pass them.

We make it to the farm and Mum pulls into a space.

"Now just try and have a nice time, darling," Mum says, her voice soft, resting her hand on my arm. "Don't push yourself too hard. It's not meant to be a competition. It's just meant to be fun."

"OK," I say, looking out of the window. Swallows swoop down from the eaves of the barns, fly low over the fields and zoom back up: flashes of scarlet, white and blue. Sparrows flit in and out of the hedgerows: little brown golf-ball-sized people who chirp.

Getting out of the car, slamming the door, I walk towards the Spin studio past the shops on my right. I can hear the music blaring out already. Suddenly, I hear a beautiful song. Looking up, I see a little sparrow singing his heart out.

"Thank you, Mr Sparrow," I say, watching him, throat open as he warbles.

Ugh, I don't want to go in here and talk to people, I think as I push open the glass door to the Spin studio. I can see a couple of people setting up their bikes and I head for my usual bike on the far left, nearest the mirrored wall, so I can see my position and only have to have a human on one side of me. Filling up my water bottles from the fountain, I adjust my saddle and handlebars. Taking a quick outfit photo for the blog in front of the mirror, I head back to my bike and climb onto it. My head is down so no one will talk to me, I hope, as I upload my outfit photo to the blog's Facebook page.

The panther lies on the floor in front of my bike. Somehow he weighs my legs down so much I can barely turn the pedals. I turn the resistance down. *I just have to get through the class*, I tell myself. The panther will affect my speed, strength and stamina. I just have to sit here throughout the class, even though every fibre of my being is screaming *run, hide, go home, lie down, die!*

Keeping my head down, hoping no one will talk to me, I start moving my legs round and adjust my red dial to resistance level three.

"Right: it's half past. Let's get going. Any injuries I should know about?" Heather the instructor says in a loud voice from her bike at the front of the class. The panther drags my ankles down with his front paws: my legs are weighted. "Can someone turn the lights down?" Heather says. Her hair is tied up in a dark brown, glossy ponytail which shines as the light hits it. She's got great hair.

"Five-minute warm-up," Heather says. "Keep the resistance low – we're warming up our legs at the moment." I can only just turn the pedals and, checking on the monitor in front of me, this is resistance level three. Pushing as hard as I can, I know it's my low mood making me feel I'm trudging through treacle and that I want to go home. Somehow knowing this doesn't make it any better.

"Standing flat," Heather says, and I stand up. "Keep the weight in the legs," she says. "Don't lean on the arms." *I want to lean on my arms*, I think. *I'm exhausted, this is torture.*

The music is so loud. The other bikes crowd my bike. I just want to step down off my bike and step out of the door into the sunlight, but I'm trapped here. *It's just another forty minutes*, I tell myself. *Forty more minutes and then I can go home and lie down for the rest of the day and cuddle my Fluffy Monster and sleep.*

"Resistance up, we're going to climb," Heather says. The music changes to a slower beat. Sitting in the saddle, pushing my legs round, I feel the change. I take a bit of resistance off: I mustn't cycle too slowly or I'll lose the beat. But I end up losing the beat anyway. Taking off yet more resistance, I find the beat. *It doesn't matter*, I tell myself as I feel the tears well up. *I'm here, that's the important thing.* But I can't stop the tears as they roll down my cheeks: tears of not being good enough. *I can always put the resistance back on when we stand*, I tell myself, feeling useless and pathetic, but surely the main thing is that I'm here, despite the panther, despite every fibre of my being screaming out in pain and despair.

"Right, take it out of the saddle," Heather says, and I stand up, put the resistance back on and push myself as hard as I can. *Soon the class will be over*, I tell myself. *I'm doing so well to be here at all.* The panther stares up at me from the floor, amber eyes wide. I know he's here to stay for a while now, and the thought fills me with foreboding and despair.

Chapter 20

OCTOBER 1997

"Cordelia, today you can help Norman with the porcupines," Derek, the head keeper of the Small Mammal House said, lengthening the 'a' in my name. Aged eighteen, I was volunteering at London Zoo in my gap year. I shuddered. Norman gave me the creeps. He was ancient: probably about thirty, swarthy with dark stubble and an earring. Yuck!

In the darkness of their enclosure, I watched the huge African brush-tailed porcupines shuffling around, their quills glowing ghostly-white in the darkness, and I was almost certain that Norman brushed against me. I pulled away, but didn't say anything. *Surely it was an accident*, I thought.

In my best friend Lily's bedroom the following evening, Thursday, we were getting ready to go clubbing at our favourite haunt, Magic Realms. I hoped that James – who I fancied – was going to be there.

"Got any silver glitter?" I asked Lily as we applied black eyeliner.

"Here you go." She handed it over. "Can you just hold this a minute?" She gave me an empty plastic bottle and started to pour vodka into it.

Walking to the station, we drank the vodka: it tasted horrible but we hadn't got much time to get wasted. Approaching the club,

I heard music pumping out into the street and recognised other Magic Realms regulars in the queue: girls from our school, boys from nearby schools, the usual bouncers. We pushed to the front – regulars got certain privileges – and with a wink to the doorman we hurtled inside like drunken fairies.

I soon encountered James. His big blue eyes made me melt: his lashes were so long. He was so vibrant and sexy, and of course so much younger and fitter than Sleazy Norman. Before long we were huddled up in a dark corner. We spent the evening kissing and drinking vodka and orange, and he promised to call me over the weekend.

The weekend came and went. James didn't call. I did the filing at my uncle's office on Monday, answered children's letters in the Zoo's Education department on Tuesday and then it was Wednesday, Small Mammal House Day. Again, I found myself assisting Norman, painting a new enclosure for the marmosets. Even though he was repulsive, I found myself telling him that I really liked James, who was older and more experienced than me and that I felt young and stupid around him.

"Don't worry, Cordelia, I'm sure you'll meet someone nice," Norman said. "Come here and give me a hug." He held out his arms and, unwillingly, I found myself hugging him. I tried to pull away, but he kept his arms round me. I broke free, feeling that sense of being trapped and a bit sick that I'd felt in the porcupine enclosure. *It's my fault*, I thought, *I shouldn't lead him on*. Resolving to keep more of a distance from him in future, I remembered Mum telling me "Men have urges, darling". I wasn't quite sure what this meant but presumed it was something to do with how important it was not to lead them on as they couldn't control themselves.

Thursday night arrived. In a dark corner of Magic Realms I was snuggled up with James. He was looking so dreamy, his dark hair grazing his cheekbones, his eyes so bright blue.

"I just need to go to the loo," I said. Once there, I reapplied my make-up.

"Hey, C, there you are," Lily said, joining me by the mirror, checking her eyeliner. She threw her arms round me. "Let's dance."

I must have spent most of the night curled up in a corner with James, kissing, giggling and talking, although I can't remember what we talked about: my memories of him now are very hazy. By the time Lily dragged me off to get the night bus, I had written my number on a piece of paper for him again ("Sorry babe, last week I put it in the back pocket of my jeans and then they went in the wash", he'd said) and again he'd promised to call me.

I spent the weekend waiting for the phone to ring, but James didn't call. Then the week unfurled: filing at my uncle's office; the cinema with Lily and then the zoo: porcupine duty again with Norman. We stood at the back of the enclosure, watching the porcupines snuffling around in the semi-dark. I felt pressure on my bum and the back of my thigh. Norman stood behind me. Moving closer, breathing more heavily, he pressed against me. I wanted to move away, yet I stayed rooted to the spot, paralysed with panic. And it was definitely deliberate that he moved closer to me. I didn't pull away. I was unable to. And we stood like that and I felt him breathing down my neck and then after what seemed like hours but could only have been a few minutes I moved away. Nothing was said, but I felt dirty and guilty. I knew I didn't want anything to happen, I knew I didn't want to be standing there with Norman touching me, but a part of me felt I was leading him on, that I deserved it.

The next day was Lily's goodbye party at Magic Realms. She was going to Israel for her whole gap year in a few days' time. I'd join her there in February, but it was only October so I'd have four months at home without her. Sitting at a table near the bar, drinking vodka and orange, I felt tired and disengaged. Lily danced with her boyfriend Geoff, who gazed at her with a soppy expression. She smiled, her eyes closed, obviously enjoying Geoff's devotion and everyone's eyes on her. Lily irritated me sometimes, but I was going to miss her.

James never even turned up that night.

At the zoo the following Wednesday I took a deep breath as I approached the Small Mammal House. If Derek tried to put me with Norman I would refuse. I had woken up feeling sick with dread and not wanting to go. As I changed into my zoo regulation uniform – brown trousers and a loose-fitting brown shirt – and tied my hair back, I knew I couldn't look much worse. My eyes were puffy from lack of sleep. There was no way I could be accused of leading Norman on, I realised. And, even if I had in some way, he was an adult, the responsible adult and, really, I was just a child.

"Ah, Cordelia, there you are," Derek said as I emerged from the changing room. "Norman's looking for you. You're late, girl, get a move on." And then he vanished down the corridor before I could say anything.

I felt my body tense up with anxiety as I went to find Norman. I stopped for a minute outside the grey slender loris enclosure. A loris was up near the glass, balancing on a branch, gazing at me with huge glowing eyes from the darkness, soft furry front legs out in front of him, his curiously truncated body poised along the branch, back legs one in front of the other and his body just stopping short, tailless. The lorises have to be kept in complete darkness: they are nocturnal forest-dwellers – very secretive and shy.

"Hello little chap," I said, looking back at him. He lifted a front leg in preparation for climbing up the branch, but it seemed as if he was waving, signalling to me. I stood there watching the exaggerated slowness of his movements as he began to climb the branch. He placed one front paw in front of the other, crossing his long legs.

Watching his curious tailless silhouette, and his long legs, I wished I could disappear inside his enclosure with him.

Once I found Norman, and we started painting the marmoset enclosure, everything seemed fine, which was puzzling. He had painted dark brown branches across the walls, and I was adding pale and darker green leaves to them. I managed to position myself on the opposite side of the enclosure, and barely said anything. With a bit of space between us the situation appeared to defuse itself.

In the afternoon, I continued adding foliage to the painted trees. Norman didn't really speak to me and we worked in peace and quiet on opposite sides of the room. I began to think I must have imagined him touching me in the weeks before.

"A young man's on the phone for you," Mum said as I opened the front door. "James, he says his name is. Who's James?"

I had to sit down with the dizzying feeling of triumph. James had called.

"Give me the phone!" I said.

"Here she is, James, she's just walked in," Mum said.

"Hello? This is Cordelia," I said.

"Hi, Cordelia. How are you doing?" he asked, sounding different on the phone, older somehow.

"OK." I said.

"Wanna meet up next Tuesday?"

"Yes," I said, trying not to sound too excited. But I was excited, James wanted to meet up with me!

"Meet you at the café at eight," he said. "Bye."

The line went dead. Next Tuesday was almost a week away. I wondered what he was doing all week. But even so, this was, at last, a date. I smiled to myself. Things were starting to improve: Norman seemed to have stopped harassing me, James was taking me on a date, I was feeling a bit more hopeful about my future.

Tuesday night arrived at last, the night of my date with James. I was really nervous: I'd never seen him outside Magic Realms before. We might have nothing to talk about in daylight, I thought. I took a swig from my bottle of vodka and a deep breath as I went inside the café.

Scanning the room, I realised James wasn't there yet. I settled down at a table in the back corner to wait. The minutes ticked by. James was fifteen minutes late. I went back to my book. After another half an hour, I realised he wasn't coming. I ran out, tears streaming down my face.

The next day, Wednesday, dawned: Small Mammal House Day. I wanted to stay in bed for days, weeks, months. I certainly didn't want to spend the day cleaning up animal droppings. I was still crying as I approached the side gate of the zoo.

Norman had been fine the previous week, but now, maybe emboldened by the increased darkness in the porcupine enclosure, he was back to his old tricks: brushing past me, touching me. Suddenly I was trapped with him in front of me and the wall behind. And then something in me snapped. Taking a deep breath I elbowed him aside, pushed past him and ran down the corridor. I didn't stop running until I was at the head keeper's office.

"Derek," I said, bursting in dishevelled, sweaty, panting. "I have to talk to you."

"Cordelia," Derek looked up from his writing. "What's the matter?"

"I have to report something," I squeezed the words out.

Derek looked puzzled.

"What do you mean? Here, take a seat." He waved towards an old sofa covered in newspaper articles, dustbin bags and old monkey gloves.

I sat down. "Norman keeps touching me."

"Are you sure?" Derek said, looking worried and perhaps sceptical, I wasn't sure.

"Well, at first I thought it was an accident," I said. "But it kept happening. And then today I just ran away, because I can't take it anymore. I'm not working with him again. I can't. He's so old and sleazy and …"

Derek let out an involuntary laugh, and then composed his face. "And how long has this been going on?"

"About six weeks," I said.

"Six whole weeks? Why didn't you say anything before now?"

"At first, I thought I might be imagining it," I said. "Then I thought it might somehow be my fault or …"

"It's not your fault. Definitely not," Derek said, shaking his head, looking concerned. "This is a serious allegation, you do realise that, Cordelia?" He looked at me, a long, searching stare.

"Yes," I said. "I know."

"For today, I want you to go and help Melissa. She's downstairs in Moonlight World. Run along now. And chin up, Cordelia. It's going to be alright." He smiled at me, a kind smile, and I felt so relieved that I wasn't going to get into trouble or be sent back into Norman's clutches.

"Hey Cordelia," Melissa said. "Do you want to go in with the bats?" I'd found her in a corridor of Moonlight World, the underground section which was very dark and full of nocturnal animals: bats, fennec foxes and echidnas.

"Yes please," I said.

"If you're very quiet," she said, "we can go in there now."

Unlocking the gate to the bat cave, Melissa pushed the heavy plastic curtains aside. I tiptoed in. At first it seemed empty, and absolutely stank. As my eyes adjusted to the light, I could see the bat droppings glistening, streaked down the walls, a pinkish white. And then I heard and felt it: hundreds of wings beating, the air waving, rippling and caressing me. The bats swooped around me, their wings brushing my face and hair in the darkness. They touched me, and I didn't mind or feel scared or trapped. Down there, in the bat cave, life held limitless possibilities.

Chapter 21

JUNE 2016

Waking up with a start, I know I don't want to be awake. *I want to die, I want to die, I want to die.* I certainly don't want to get up. The panther lies on top of me, crushing the breath out of my body. But I haul myself out of bed, somehow, and crawl through to the kitchen in my flat to make breakfast. Pouring some milk into my porridge, I put it in the microwave for two and a half minutes, boil the kettle and make a cup of coffee. When the microwave pings I cut a banana into slices and place them on the top of my porridge and squeeze some golden syrup in swirls on the banana.

Taking my breakfast back into my bedroom, I arrange the pillows behind me so I can sit up with my back against the headboard.

Putting Absolute Radio 90s on, I attempt to drown out my dark thoughts with the sounds of Christian and Richie talking.

"It's no wonder Seb left you," the panther says. "You're fat and useless and infertile. You're no good to anyone."

This seems incontrovertible. I focus on dressing: socks then knickers and vest top. My implants stand up on their own so I no longer need a bra, which is good. It looks warm out there: checking my phone it says twenty-two degrees, so I put on my fuchsia-pink knee-length cotton dress and some FitFlops. Cleaning my teeth, wiping my face, spraying some Chanel Coco

Mademoiselle, I put on a cotton hairband and pick up a pink cardigan, putting it in my bag.

In the kitchen I pick up two slices of bread, a couple of carrots, an apple, a cereal bar, a can of Diet Coke and a banana and put them in my bag. Walking to the bus stop past trees white with apple blossom and pink with cherry blossom, I wait for my bus.

"You're back," my colleague says when I arrive at the office, an authors' and actors' agency. "It's so good to see you. How are you?" She smiles at me, and we have a hug.

"I'm OK," I say, not wanting to tell her about Seb just yet. I know if I can just focus on my work it will make me feel better, so I print out all the castings from the website and scrawl on them in pencil which of our actors I think would be right for certain roles, leaving these on my boss's desk for her to check.

"How good to see you," my boss says when she arrives.

"Would you like a cup of tea?" I ask her.

"Yes, why not, and a biscuit please," she says.

I make her tea how she likes it: weak with no milk and carry it through with the biscuit tin. It feels better to be amongst other people, doing something other than thinking about my physical or mental health or my broken heart. Sitting with my boss whilst she does the castings, I look at the posters on her walls of past productions of our plays and, behind her, books by our long-dead authors. She scribbles out my suggestions with a pencil and writes her own ideas, brow furrowed with concentration.

"All done," she says to me, and I take them into the next room, where I input the suggestions on the casting website. As I complete each one, I write the date in red biro on the top right-hand corner of the page and put it into a basket.

Phone calls come in: people wanting to speak to my boss, casting directors offering appointments for actors. I call the actors, tell them where to go and when, whether they need to prepare a song and if so in what style, what they need to wear. Sometimes I tell them that there are some pages which will be emailed and that I will forward them on.

At lunch time, I take my sandwiches to the little park near the office. Alcoholics sit on the benches round the sides of the park, drinking their cans of Stella and Fosters. Ignoring them, I look at the palm trees and pretty tropical vegetation that has been planted in an effort to clean up the junkie park. The panther stretches out next to me but I ignore him and watch the pigeons striding around, heads bobbing, and the blackbirds who pull worms out of the earth with yellow beaks.

I lie on my front on top of my cardigan on a gentle slope in the park when I've finished my lunch. It's sunny now and my legs are exposed – *I'll feel better if I can get a bit of a tan*, I think.

"You're so fat," the panther says, staring at me with amber eyes. "And that dress really doesn't suit you – you really ought to make more of an effort with your appearance. You're not young anymore, you know. You're thirty-seven. The clock is ticking."

Trying to ignore him, I realise tears are running down my cheeks.

"How are you feeling, Cordelia?" my psychiatrist Dr Stein asks me as we sit in his office the following week. I've been seeing him for years now, eighteen years, ever since I was first diagnosed with cyclothymia, the embryonic form of bipolar I became ill with at university.

"Well, my mood is still low," I say. "It's been low for three months now and …"

"And do you want to do anything about that, Cordelia? You know what I've told you several times already," Dr Stein says, sounding resigned. "You could try quetiapine. There are some extremely persuasive new results that it is the best treatment for your form of the illness, one with recurrent depressive episodes. I heard a paper about it at the Royal

College of Psychiatrists last week. A combination of quetiapine and sodium valproate seems to be the most effective treatment for people who suffer mostly from depressive episodes and …"

"I'm not taking that stuff," I say.

"Why not?" Dr Stein puts his head on one side, fixing me with his blue-eyed stare.

"Because everyone I know who takes quetiapine is obese. I'm not prepared to put on six stone or …"

"I have plenty of patients who take it who aren't obese," Dr Stein says, smiling. I flatter myself that he finds me amusing, that I'm a welcome break from his other patients, who I imagine to be humourless, antipsychotic-bloated, flabby creatures.

"Well, I'm sorry, but I'm not taking it," I say, shaking my head.

"It's up to you, Cordelia," he says. "I can't make you take it, but I have a duty of care towards you, and if I don't tell you about alternative medication options I'm not doing my job properly."

"People who I know who take that drug can't stop eating. One girl I know described how she sits there in a quetiapine-induced stupor, shovelling cereal into her mouth. I know those antipsychotics do something to your metabolism," I say.

"Fine. We'll leave your medication how it is. How's everything else?" Dr Stein asks me – pen poised above the paper.

The panther sits on the floor next to my chair. He has a difficult relationship with Dr Stein: his hackles are up and he's growling. Sometimes I think he regards Dr Stein as a threat, but I'm probably just being stupid.

"Things are OK," I say.

"Are you socialising?" He starts writing something in my notes. I wonder what it is. I can't quite see from the other side of the desk.

"A bit," I say, even though I'm not.

"How's your appetite?"

"OK," I say, although if I didn't drink a couple of glasses of wine with every meal I doubt I'd be able to eat much: I'm not hungry at the moment but I know I have to eat to keep my strength up.

"How's work?"

"It's fine," I say, even though it's not.

"Are you creating opportunities to meet new people?" he asks, his eyes full of concern.

"Yes," I say, even though I haven't seen anyone except my ex-flatmate Suzy and my work colleagues and my parents for months. *I feel hollowed out by the end of my relationship with Seb*, I think, as I start to pull the skin from my thumbs. I've been dealing with this illness since I was nineteen, for eighteen years. It's too long. I know I should have made some more progress by now. Blood pours from my thumbs where I've ripped the skin. The panther licks the wounds.

"Are you still meditating?" Dr Stein asks. I started meditating a few years ago now, and whilst my mood was up it seemed to help, it seemed to relax me. But now it doesn't seem to be helping anymore.

"Yes," I say. "Twice a day: before my afternoon sleep and before I go to sleep at night."

"Maybe that will help your low mood," Dr Stein says. "I think we should leave your medication where it is, I don't want to change anything. Do you want to ask your mother if she would like to come in for a bit?" Dr Stein asks me.

I go out into the corridor. "Mum, Dr Stein would like you to come in," I tell her.

Mum puts down her half-finished *The Times* crossword and follows me into Dr Stein's office, her heels making a decisive clicking sound on the floor.

"Hello, Dr Stein," Mum says, smoothing her hair and smiling at him. She sits in the chair next to mine and pulls it closer to the desk, nearer to Dr Stein. She's always had a bit of a crush on him.

"Hello, Mrs Feldman. I was just wondering how Cordelia is at the moment, from your point of view."

"She's still a bit miserable," Mum says. "It does seem to go on for such a long time these days. And we're worried that she doesn't seem to want to go out with people her own age – she seems to want to spend all her time with us and …"

"That's not true, Mum," I say. "I went out for dinner with Suzy on Tuesday and …"

"You know that isn't what I mean, Cordelia," Mum says, shaking her head. "I just don't want Cordelia to be on her own, Dr Stein, after we are gone and …"

"Mum, please stop it," I say. "You're not helping."

"Dr Stein, I just don't know why she can't meet a nice Jewish boy and settle down," Mum says.

Dr Josh looks from Mum to me and then back to Mum.

"I am sure Cordelia will meet someone when she is ready, Mrs Feldman," he says.

"But how, if she spends all her time with us?" Mum asks.

"That's not true Mum, I went to that event at the zoo with Suzy and Gemma and …"

"That was in April, Cordelia," Mum says. "It is now June, and I don't think you've been to a social event since then."

"Cordelia, will you make a real effort to go to some social events please?" Dr Stein asks. "The key to a successful single social life is planning, and you need to make plans, at least two or three times a week, to meet new people. We have talked about this before."

"Yes, Dr Stein," I say.

"Good. I'll see you in a month. Look after yourselves, both of you," he says opening the door for us, ushering us out.

"Thank you, Dr Stein." Mum says, smiling at him.

"Thank you," I say, mustering up a smile of my own.

We walk to the car.

"I don't know why you have to be so … why do you have to talk about me with Dr Stein like I'm a small child," I say to Mum, feeling irritated and unfortunately sounding irritable.

"I just worry about you, darling" Mum says, her voice softened. "I'm always going to be your mother, Cordelia."

"I know, I'm sorry Mum. I know you're just trying to help," I say, putting my arm round her.

Chapter 22

I remember the first time I clapped eyes on Seb, in 2005. He was loping down the Portobello Road in front of me – his faded baggy jeans hanging off his hips, his tight grey t-shirt clinging to his body – and I thought "I'll die if I don't have him," so I engaged him in conversation. He was even more beautiful from the front: my fantasy made flesh and just dropped in the road in front of me. I was twenty-six and he was twenty-four then. I was on my lunchbreak from work at the agency, where I worked for nigh on fifteen years.

The memories come thick and fast: having sex in his basement flat in Leamington Road Villas. We had to move the double mattress in from the empty room and drag it onto the bed – throwing those scarves from Morocco on top of the bare mattress because, of course, there weren't any sheets. On our first date, kissing for hours in the Bed Bar; kissing in Osteria Basilico during dinner with, as I remember him saying, a "supersonic kissing sound." We always did lots of kissing. And other things: the first night we slept together, after his play – oh that three-quarter length grey frock coat and those riding boots, how could I not – when he turned the light on to look at my piercings and then, when we were shagging, him saying "I really want to come all over you". I remember drinking and playing Would You Rather and the next day when we woke up he said: "I wouldn't do it with James Dean. I didn't mean it, I was drunk." And the time he got chilli in my minge. I think of him chopping chillies, bending over the wooden chopping board – tiny pieces, painstaking concentration. He always had that attention to detail – baking bread, learning lines, hours of ballet to play Nijinsky in the Faun thing.

"I want you to feel what I feel" I remember crying to him when he split up with me, the first or was it second time.

And then when we were together again before he went into the monastery – four years after our first stab at a relationship. At the bus stop I leant into Seb and turned my face into his chest. Our breathing quickened. We stood like this for a minute and then the tears were running down my cheeks unbidden and I turned my face up to his and closed my eyes and he kissed me and his eyes were closed and he pushed his leg in between my thighs and then I broke away.

"You don't want to be doing this, do you?" I asked, thinking about all the things Seb had been saying earlier about not wanting to do any sexual misconduct, the definition of which is fluid.

"No, sorry," he said, looking embarrassed. "No, I mean I do, but I don't."

"Is it sexual misconduct if it means something to me?" I asked.

"Um, well," he looked shifty, and uncomfortable.

"Because I really like you and if we do anything, then it means something."

He looked awkward, and fixed his eyes on a point far away, behind my head. And, no doubt, turned his thoughts to the Far East (Java, where he'd just been) or Warwickshire, the location of his monastery, near Coventry.

"I really like you. I always did." I broke off and looked into his eyes which were deep-set and half-closed in the moonlight. In the light they were turquoise. "I want to be with you," I said. "I want to spend this time with you before you go into the monastery." I was crying now. I'd been drinking, three glasses of wine to his none. Since he took his precepts he hadn't been drinking so I was drinking for both of us. I was feeling these waves of lust and I didn't know what he was feeling.

"I don't want you to be upset," he said.

"I'm upset anyway," I said, and then I was kissing him, or he was kissing me, I didn't know who started it but we were reaching for each other in the dark and we were kissing like animals that hadn't eaten for a very long time. "I'm going to be upset anyway. Why shouldn't I have something nice in my life? I've been so unhappy."

"Let's not do it if it's going to upset you," he said.

"I want to spend this time with you," I said, holding on to him. "When can I see you?"

"At the weekend. We can go for a walk on Hampstead Heath."

"We were meant to be together," I said. "Out of all your ex-girlfriends, you found me."

"I found you by accident," he said, surprised, I thought.

I leant into him, tears running down my cheeks…

I still hold the picture in my mind of his tongue lapping against me, my hands tangled in his thick dirty blond hair, and the feeling of his tongue inside me. I loved sucking his cock and licking his balls and feeling his cock swell in my mouth. I loved the taste of him and the feel of his velvety skin next to mine and how hard he held me to him, his beautiful arms wrapped around me: so strong, muscles rippling. I still love him.

I just want to hold him, kiss him, touch him, be close to him and hear his voice. I know this time, unlike all the other times, it really is over. I want to see his face again. I never dreamt I would feel such happiness and then have it ripped from me. I want to wrap my arms round him, protect him, and shelter him with a love and stability he's never known. I want to fix him. And I want him to fix me. In my mind, I kiss his smooth shoulders and all down his stomach and I stroke up his thighs and my heart rises in my throat and it's going to burst.

I remember walking around Hyde Park with Seb, walking through the empty park at night with the bats flitting around us, walking around the lake. Trekking through the woods on Hampstead Heath and then suddenly coming across that pagoda rising out of the trees. All the days I spent with Seb are suffused with sunlight and laughter and sprinkles of magic. All the time I spent with him is so precious: watching the deer at Golders Hill Park; those white silky chickens running towards us and squawking and Seb making perfect clucking noises back at them – all that acting training was useful for something. I remember all those tense goodbyes, holding each other, at stations and bus stops; imbued with the will-we-wont-we as we held onto each other. Brushing my cheek against his, breathing in his essence. Watching him take photographs of trees he liked with the enchantment of a child discovering the world.

And now he is gone forever, and I don't know how I'm going to live without him, I think, the tears rolling down my cheeks. He'd told me this time, he said "I'll stay with you till the end". But I'm still alive and I've lost the love of my life and I don't want to go on living without him.

Chapter 23

"I want to stop drinking," I say to Dr Stein. We're sitting in his consulting room. It's August now – I split up with Seb in March. The panther lies on the floor at my feet, dozing, his chin resting on his front paws. Every so often he twitches an ear or his whiskers in his sleep.

"How did it go when you last attempted to cut down your drinking?" he asks, gazing at me with his piercing blue eyes, pen poised above my notes.

"I tried, but I just couldn't manage it," I say. "I'm having my first gin and Slimline tonic at about eleven thirty in the morning on days when I'm not at work and I'm twitching and agitated until I can get a drink and I just feel I'm a slave to it now. At least when I was with Seb we were drinking together, now I'm drinking on my own when I'm at the flat and …"

"How much do you estimate you're drinking?" Dr Stein asks, his voice full of concern.

"About a bottle of wine per day," I say. "Or half a bottle of gin. And since I changed from carbamazepine to lurasidone I'm so anxious and …"

"The alcohol withdrawal is causing the anxiety," he says. "The carbamazepine dampened that down since it's a sedative, but since lurasidone isn't a sedative you're experiencing the alcohol withdrawal, before your first drink of the day, as anxiety."

"Oh," I say.

"Also, with the amount you're drinking it's a risk to put you under general anaesthetic without prescribing Librium for you," he says.

This all sounds much more serious than I thought, I think.

"What's Librium?" I ask.

"It's a benzodiazepine," he says. "I'll put you on it and we'll do something called a phased withdrawal where we start cutting down the dose straight away. You'll be recuperating at your parents' house so you'll be safe. The phased withdrawal will take about ten days and after that we'll maintain you on clonazepam. Does that sound sensible?"

"Yes," I say. "Can I get Dad now?"

"Of course," Dr Stein says, scribbling in my notes.

I go out into the corridor. Dad is reading the *Financial Times*. He's hidden behind the salmon-pink broadsheet.

"Dad," I say. "You can come in now."

"Jolly good," Dad says, getting up, folding his paper.

"So," Dr Stein says, once Dad and I are settled on the other side of his desk. "We've been talking about your daughter's drinking and it seems she has developed an alcohol problem."

"I'm surprised," Dad says. "I know she likes a drink but I hadn't realised she has a problem." He looks at me and it breaks my heart because he looks so disappointed in me.

"I'm afraid she does," Dr Stein says, sounding sympathetic.

This is so humiliating, I think. The panther glares at me from the floor. "You're so pathetic," he says, amber eyes wide with disgust. "You're such a disappointment to your father. Tears are running down my cheeks.

"I'm so sorry, Dad," I say, not even able to bring myself to look at him, I'm so full of self-loathing. I don't even know when my drinking went from a social thing, the same as other people's drinking, to this. *I'm a slave to alcohol and I can't live like this any longer*, I think.

"We're going to get you through this," Dr Stein says. "So, sir, as I was explaining to your daughter just before, with the amount she's drinking it would be dangerous to put her under a general anaesthetic as she'll go into withdrawal and …"

"I had no idea," Dad says, sounding shocked, shaking his head. Suddenly he looks so old and helpless sitting there, grey-haired, wrinkled, exhausted. *I've done this to him*, I think, hating myself.

"What I'm going to do is when she goes in for her surgery I'm going to prescribe her Librium and that has a phased withdrawal," Dr Stein says. "The withdrawal will be started in hospital but once she's home, you or your wife will give her the exact amounts specified and …"

"Will it stop her craving alcohol?" Dad asks.

"Yes, it will. And the plan is gradually to cut the Librium down to nothing over about ten days and to maintain her on clonazepam after that. The carbamazepine is a sedative you see, so it dampens down the anxiety caused by daily alcohol withdrawal. Now she's on lurasidone which isn't a sedative, she needs an anti-anxiety drug as well."

"I see," Dad says, looking at me. "I had no idea things were this bad – I thought she just liked a drink and …"

"I'm afraid it's far more serious than that," Dr Stein says. "Your daughter tells me that she's tried and failed to reduce her alcohol intake and …"

"So, this Librium stuff works, does it?" Dad says.

"Yes, sir. It's a good treatment," Dr Stein says. "So, I'll see you after your operation," he says, looking at me. "I'll sort out prescriptions for the Librium and the clonazepam with the pharmacy here," he says.

"Thank you," I say, getting up.

"Take care of yourself," he says to me. "Goodbye, sir," he says to Dad.

"Thank you very much, Dr Stein," Dad says, as they shake hands.

I'm in the antechamber in front of the operating theatre. It's just big enough for me, lying down on a bed, and the anaesthetist and a nurse.

"Are you allergic to anything?" the anaesthetist asks.

"Most kinds of plasters and dressings," I say. "Except the pink Micropore and Elastoplast."

"How about this one?" he asks, holding up a plastic Tegaderm dressing.

"Yes, I'm allergic to that one, sorry," I say. "Oh, and I can't have injections in either arm because I've had all my nodes out."

"OK," the anaesthetist says, pushing his glasses up to the bridge of his nose. "We'll put the cannula in your foot then."

"My foot will get cold," I say.

"Very soon you'll be unconscious," he says.

Wincing with pain as the cannula is inserted into my foot, I start to look forward to the general anaesthetic and being deeply asleep.

"Now, you'll feel something cold, that's the anaesthetic going in," the anaesthetist says.

A very cold liquid enters my vein from the cannula.

"One, two, three, four," he says. And then there's nothing.

I'll spare you the coming-round-after-the-operation bit because I've already described that earlier in the book. Suffice to say, I wake up and am, after a decent interval, wheeled back to my room. I have drains in and I'm on morphine. Lying in my hospital room, I watch *Top Gear* repeats and wait for Mum to arrive.

The door opens.

"Mum," I croak, my mouth dry from the operation.

"Hello, darling," Mum says, crossing the room to sit in the chair next to me. Stroking my hair, she takes hold of my hand. "I'm here now, I'll look after you, it's going to be OK."

"Mum, I need the loo," I say.

"OK darling," Mum says. We detach my drain bottles from the sides of the bed and put them in a plastic bag. Sitting up slowly, I lean on Mum as I swing my legs around and lower my feet to the floor. Straightening up, I lean on Mum's shoulder and she holds me as I walk the three steps to the bathroom. Lowering myself down onto the loo, I pull down my knitted hospital pants. A gush of wee comes out. No poo: the morphine is constipating. Standing up, leaning on Mum, I hobble to the sink, turn the taps on. Washing my hands, I catch a glimpse of myself in the mirror. I'm so pale.

"I look awful," I say to Mum.

"You've just had major surgery, darling," Mum says, helping me back to bed. She takes the drain bottles from me and fastens one to each side of the bed frame.

"I'm thirsty," I say.

Mum pours me some water from the jug and puts it on my bedside table.

"My chest hurts," I say. Looking down at my chest I can see bandages. I wonder what it looks like underneath. This is the operation where finally I've been given my silicone implants: replacing my saline ones. This is not as major as some of my operations have been but still: I've had general anaesthetic, I have drains and I'm all bandaged up.

After a while there's a knock on the door.

"Hi, I've brought you your sandwich," the girl says. She's wearing black with a white frilly apron over it. I haven't eaten since the night before – many, many hours ago.

"Thank you," I say. As I start eating my sandwich I realise how starving I am. *Well done me*, I think. *I've survived yet another operation. I haven't started needing a drink yet, so that's good – must be the effect of the Librium.* I start to feel really tired.

"Mum, I'm just going to have a sleep I think," I say, pushing my table away, pressing the button to lower the head of my bed.

"OK darling," Mum says. "I'll sit here and do the crossword."

"Thank you for staying with me, Mum," I say, taking Mum's hand. "I love you."

"I love you too, my darling," Mum says, stroking my hand

In hospital my days are regimented and it's the best place to be right now. Now the panther's here, I sleep through till eight o'clock in the morning when the nurse comes to take my blood pressure, mark on my drain bottles to show how much new fluid has accumulated in each bottle overnight and give me my morning medication in a little waxed paper cup. Then breakfast arrives and I can watch a film on one of the movie channels. I watch *Fly Away Home* starring a young Anna Paquin as a girl who has lost her mother and raises a flock of greylag geese and flies them on migration. Mum arrives at about nine o'clock – after she's had her own breakfast – and we watch *Top Gear* or *Wild at Heart* – a series about a vet and his family who have a surgery and co-own a game reserve in South Africa. It stars Stephen Tompkinson and features Hayley Mills as the wife of the alcoholic South African game reserve owner, Du Plessis. There are, of course, lions and elephants and giraffes and so on and the series is great fun.

Mum leaves after lunch and I have my sleep and then wake up and watch *Poirot* or *Marple* until Dad arrives at about six o'clock, when it's supper time. We watch a film and then Dad leaves and I go to sleep after my night-time medication.

So, it's a regimented but low-stress time. The morphine keeps me in a dreamlike state. Nothing is required of me. I have no visitors apart from my parents. It's welcome respite from my real life. I'm happy in hospital – the morphine keeps the panther quiet.

"We're going to take these drains out and then you can go home," the nurse says on the morning of the sixth day. "Hardly any fluid is coming out now and …"

"Can I have some Oramorph?" I ask, remembering how painful drain-removal can be.

"I'll just get you some Oramorph and then we'll wait thirty minutes or so for it to take effect," the nurse says, marking on each of my three drain bottles how much fluid has arrived during the night. It isn't more than ten millilitres or so in each bottle.

She leaves the room. I look out of the window at the trees. The leaves are turning yellow and red and orange. It's early September – the beginning of autumn. I came in here at the end of August, in the last days of summer. *I hope there will be a few more sunny days once I'm home*, I think. I find autumn difficult: the beginning of nature's process of decay, the shortening days and the increasing darkness. I've never really lost that back-to-school feeling and each autumn I wish I'm starting another degree, but it's been more than ten years since I started my creative writing master's in 2005 – it's now 2016. And I haven't published a novel in that time.

"Here you go, swallow this," the nurse says, returning with a tiny, waxed paper cup of Oramorph. I swallow the sweet liquid and she leaves me. Picking up the phone I dial my parental home.

"Hello," Mum answers.

"Mum," I say, "it's me."

"Hello, darling," Mum says. "How are you this morning?"

"They're going to take my drains out so I can come home," I say. "So can you come and get me?"

"I'll be with you in about an hour and a half then, darling," Mum says. "You know it always takes them a while to pack up your pills for discharge and so on."

"I'll see you soon," I say.

"See you in about an hour and a half then," Mum says. "I don't want you to pack anything up in case you hurt yourself – I'll do it when I arrive."

"OK, I won't," I say. "Bye Mum."

"Bye, darling," Mum says. "Your pussycat will be so pleased to see you." Her voice softens as she talks about darling Fluffball.

"How is he?" I ask. "I've missed him so much."

"He was fine at seven o'clock this morning when he went out without his breakfast," Mum says. "He'll probably be coming in for a mid-morning snack at about the time we get home."

"I can't wait to see him," I say. "See you soon."

Putting the phone down, I wait for the nurses to come back and remove my drains. It will be nice to see my Spitfire. I've missed cuddling him. But it will be difficult in some ways to be helpless at my parental home. I'll get meals cooked for me but I won't have the privacy I have here, or a television in my bedroom. I'll have to lie on the sofa in the living room in the middle of the open-plan house, whilst my parents scurry around after me. Rather than spending their retirement on cruise ships and taking their grandchildren on days out, as all their friends do, they look after me and ferry me to and from hospital appointments, scans and to see my psychiatrist.

Even though it's not my fault, I can't help feeling a sense of guilt that their lives are so miserable. I'm shielded from some of my miseries by the very fact that my mood is up for about 60 per cent of the time. But they have to be vigilant: whether my mood is high or low, they worry about me all the time.

The morphine kicks in. I start to float and my cares drift away. *Ah, that's better*, I think, smiling, as I wait for the nurses to return, wait for discharge, caught in a state of suspended animation.

Watching the clouds drift across the sky, I'm floating with them, free from this earthly body that's given me so much trouble. My spirit soars unshackled above the trees.

Chapter 24

At home, my parents start to taper off my Librium and when it's finished I start on the clonazepam. I'm still on codeine for the pain too, so I'm not quite back to reality, but for the first time since my cancer diagnosis I'm Not Drinking.

I've had a couple of previous alcohol-free periods: one when I first left the mental hospital aged twenty-six and one aged thirty-one for about four months before I went to Florence to do a three month history of art and Italian course. After both of those dry periods, I went back to drinking with renewed fervour. But this time it's different. This time it's going to be for good. At least, that's the plan.

Drinking has shaped my whole adult life, since I was about fifteen. I've had periods where I've been drinking more than others but it's been a constant crutch. I've always had a couple of glasses of wine with supper, always drunk at parties. And now, I'm not just single but sober. I'm not back at work yet and my life is blank.

I go to Spin every morning and other than that I go for walks and watch television and write the blog and that's it. My parents take care not to drink in front of me. It's so boring: not drinking, being sober.

Alcohol made me forget. Brick in Tennessee Williams' *Cat on a Hot Tin Roof,* – which I studied for English A-level – describes a "click" when he becomes drunk enough and towards the end of my drinking life I too was drinking until I felt a click where everything

159

felt OK until I passed out. Now I'm just here, with my feelings: the panther and missing Seb and, generally, what a mess everything is.

Stopping drinking is meant to be giving me back control but it doesn't feel like that somehow. It just feels dull. Now I have nothing to look forward to, no time of the day when anything will feel better. Waking up with a sort-of clear head is good up to a point, but I'm still depressed, heartbroken and in pain.

"It's so boring," I say to Mum, as I sit at the table one evening. It's supper time.

"Eat your food," Mum says.

Looking at my Quorn and mushrooms in tomato sauce and baked potato and purple sprouting broccoli, I shake my head. "I'm not hungry," I say.

"You have to eat your supper," Mum says. "Just eat some of the Quorn and a bit of the potato and …"

"I don't have any appetite without alcohol," I say, spearing a piece of purple sprouting broccoli on my fork, putting it in my mouth, chewing it. "I just can't enjoy my food without wine," I say.

"I'm so sorry," Mum says, sounding sad. "I don't see why you can't just drink like a normal person and …"

"Because I have an alcohol problem," I say. "If I could just drink a normal amount then I would, but I can't."

"I still don't understand why," Mum says.

"It's probably something to do with my mental disorder," I say. "There's a high rate of co-morbidity between manic depression and addiction – about 50 per cent, you know."

"I just feel sorry for you darling," Mum says. "Not being able to have a drink or …"

"I feel sorry for myself too," I say. Forcing down some of the Quorn mixture, I put my knife and fork down. "Can I have a chocolate please?" I ask.

"Of course you can, sweetie, they're in the fridge," Mum says.

Taking my plate through to the kitchen, I put it and my knife and fork in the dishwasher. Opening the fridge, I see the box of chocolates on a shelf about halfway down and pick it up and take it through to the dining room.

"Since I've stopped drinking I've started craving chocolate all the time." I say to my parents.

"Just goes to show it's also the sugar you're addicted to," Dad says.

"Maybe I'll lose some of the weight I've put on with the cancer treatment," I say, sipping my sparkling water with lemon squash, which I take as strong as possible.

"I'm sure you will," Mum says, with conviction. "You're eating much less than you were before and of course you're not consuming all those empty alcohol calories."

"I'm just not hungry," I say. "And eating just isn't enjoyable without being able to wash my food down with a glass of wine. And I always lose my appetite when I'm depressed."

"Maybe you won't be depressed for too long this time," Mum says.

"After all," Dad says. "Alcohol is a depressant and now you're not drinking …"

"Well, I've still got a mood cycle," I say. "And I've changed drugs and I don't know how long it's going to take for the lurasidone to work or if I'm even at a therapeutic dose or …"

"Let's just hope you're not depressed for that long this time then," Mum says, picking up her and Dad's plates. I pick up the round white ceramic bowl which had contained the vegetables, and take it into the kitchen. Refilling my glass of lemon squash and sparkling water, I take it downstairs to the living room. Spitfire is on his pink chair, head resting on his front paws, long feathery tail hanging down. He dozes. I stroke him gently on the top of his head, and he stretches his neck, waking up. Stroking him under the chin, I listen to his purr. *It's going to be OK*, I think. *I'm here with my parents and my cat who love me, my mood will come up, I'll stop wanting to drink. Things will get better.* Turning the television on, I find an episode of *Midsomer Murders* in the recordings' library.

"Can we watch *Midsomer Murders*?" I ask.

"Of course we can," Mum says, coming down the stairs, sitting next to me on the sofa. "Come on," she says to Dad, who is still at the table.

Dad comes down the stairs into the living room and settles himself into his chair. Then we're transported to Midsomer, where there's a pet show on and a prize rabbit has disappeared. Curling my legs underneath me on the sofa, I settle in and prepare for murder to be committed …

"It's no wonder Seb dumped you," the panther says. I've just woken up from my afternoon sleep and he's lying on top of me, pressing me down into the mattress. His breath smells of rotting meat – it's horrible. "You're so fat," he says.

He's right: I've put on twenty-two pounds with the cancer treatment.

"I know," I say. "But now you're here and I'm not drinking, the weight will come off. Or some of it will. It's bound to." Attempting to sit up, I push the panther off me. Lying next to me in my bed, he turns away from me and starts grooming his flank.

Pulling on my pyjama trousers, I slide my feet into some FitFlops and put a pink fleece over my top half. "Come on, we're going for a walk," I say, opening my bedroom door.

My parents are sitting in the living room. Mum is doing *The Times* crossword. Lips pursed in concentration, she's put some letters in a lump on a blank bit of page and is looking at them. It must be an anagram. Dad is dozing in his chair.

"Just going for a walk round the block," I say.

"OK, sweetie," Mum says. "What would you like for supper?"

"A scrambled egg please," I say.

"I'll make you a scrambled egg with cheese and mushrooms then," Mum says, writing the letters into the crossword: anagram solved.

"Thank you, Mum," I say. "Where's my Fluffy?"

"Still out," Mum says. "Make sure you look behind you to see if he's following you down the road."

"Yes, I will," I say. Sometimes the Fluffy Monster follows Mum down our road, across the next road and into a nearby road, which is not to be encouraged. Sometimes he lies down in the middle of the road for a rest, the fluffy fool.

Outside, I can't be bothered to walk round the block, but I force myself. The panther pads beside me on huge paws. Looking back, I don't see Spitfire, so that's good.

My parents' road is a crescent that joins the nearest road at both ends. I head right out of the house and then turn left at the end of the road. Going this way round the walk ensures I get the uphill bit out of the way at the beginning so on the way back I'll be heading downhill. There's a gorgeous little rockery at the end of my parents' road which I pass. There are no cars out on the road but a grey squirrel bounds across and into the hedge. Sometimes I see a local dog-walker I know, Hayley, or one of the neighbours, but I don't see anyone today.

Towards the far end of the road there are cedar trees which drop cones. It's pleasurable walking on the softened dropped needles and walking beneath the cedar trees which reach high up into the sky. At the end I turn left, back into the far end of our road. I pass the entrance to the woods but don't go in, although it's a beautiful walk through them. Today I'm just doing the fifteen minute circuit round the block. The sky presses down on me and it's an effort to move my feet: walking through treacle. The panther pads beside me.

It's September now which means he's been with me for six months which is the longest time we've ever been together.

"It's time for you to go," I say to him.

"I like it here, with you," he says, glaring at me with amber eyes. "You haven't got anyone else to be with you, now Seb's gone and he's never coming back."

"I've got my parents, and Spitfire," I say, as we enter our end of the road. In about five minutes' time we'll be home and I'd better have a bath – it's been a few days but whilst the panther's here I don't feel like taking my clothes off and getting wet and having to dry myself and dress again. It's too much effort.

Approaching my parental home, I check under the cars to see if Spitfire is about. Near the front door I see him sitting in front of it, fluffy tail curled round his paws. I pick him up, he feels so heavy as he goes limp in my arms – a Ragdoll trait.

Carrying him into his bedroom, I pour out some food for him. He dives into it, and I hear a loud crunching as I leave him in his room.

"Spitfire's in," I say to Mum as I enter the kitchen and walk past her to the side door to close the cat flap.

"Will you close the back door then?" Mum asks. She is frying some mushrooms for my scrambled egg.

"Yes, OK," I say. "I'm going to have a bath."

"Good idea," Mum says.

In the bathroom, I run my bath and pour some Simple foam into it as I'm allergic to everything else. Taking off my clothes, I sit in the bath. It's too hot so I put a bit of cold water in until the temperature feels right. Turning onto my front, I tie my hair up so it doesn't get wet. Now it's six o'clock, my mood has started to lift as it does every evening around this time. I'm looking forward to supper and to watching television and then going to sleep. *Maybe when I wake up in the morning the panther will have gone*, I think, as I soak in the bubbles.

Chapter 25

Having secondary breast cancer has taught me some things which I'm going to share with you now. When I was first diagnosed, I was devastated that I had breast cancer to deal with on top of my bipolar 1 disorder, because I'd already learnt about pushing myself to go to work when I don't feel like it, the importance of exercise and the vital urgency of spending some time in nature and with animals. As well as, of course, about trying to avoid stress, learning to say no and not pushing myself too hard – by the time my breast cancer diagnosis arrived I'd been working part-time and exercising about five times a week for almost my whole adult life. But no matter, I had been chosen by G-d to have a chronic terminal illness on top of my chronic mental disorder.

Things That Having Secondary Breast Cancer Has Taught Me

- Keep working if you possibly can. I carried on working part-time during chemotherapy and whenever I could between treatments, and that really helped me for the first few years after my cancer diagnosis. I don't feel well enough to go to work now, but I kept attending the office for as long as I could so I had something to think about other than my physical and mental health. I kept a connection with the world and other people and felt a sense of achievement.

- Seize the day. You know all those things you've been putting off? Just do them. For example, Mum didn't want to take me to Venice as she thought I should go with my husband, but I haven't acquired a husband yet, so I went to Venice with Mum and it was wonderful. Or, if there's a course you've always wanted to do, do it. I did tarot, advanced tarot and am now doing a three-year astrology diploma that will allow me to be an accredited astrologer. Or if there's someone for whom you have feelings, tell them. Once I found out I had breast cancer, I realised that I had a love of my life, Seb, and I was going to persuade him to meet me. It took about another eighteen months for me to make him my boyfriend, and the relationship ended, of course, but at least I know I did everything in my power to have a relationship with him.

- Friendships. When someone is diagnosed with a serious illness, the balance of friendships change. I've found some of my friends have been brilliant, others pretty useless, and some surprising people have been wonderful. I've had to let some things go in order to hold onto some old friends who I really don't want to lose. I've ended up valuing certain friends even more and letting go of some others who were toxic friends, such as the aforementioned Lily.

- Family. Some people in your family will be wonderful, others less so. I'm so grateful to my long-suffering parents and amazing brother who have looked after me so well, and special mention goes to my cousin Patrick's wife Julia who met me when I was having chemotherapy and has been such a source of strength and friendship throughout all my treatment.

- Exercise. It will improve outcomes so the fitter you are the better, I think. I have kept exercising all the way through my treatments: going to the gym every day before radiotherapy, going to Spin three or four or five times per week. Since about a year after diagnosis, I've been seeing a personal trainer once a week. She helps me to lift weights safely. She knows all the treatment I've had and pushes me far harder than I push myself. If the gym is not for you, then walking and swimming are great exercise, or joining a tennis club or netball team. The important thing is to find an exercise you love and commit to it. Now I do Pilates three times per week and have taken up barre, a ballet and Pilates fusion, twice a week.

- You don't have to be positive. All that stuff about being positive is rubbish. If you've just been diagnosed with a life-threatening illness it's OK to be scared. If all you can do is watch television, that's OK too. You don't have to be anything. It's perfectly understandable to mourn for your old life and to feel devastated. You will move on and come to terms with it, but it's natural not to feel positive about things and that's perfectly acceptable.

- Eat what you want. Don't be taken in by this-food-causes-cancer or this-food-prevents-cancer. If that were true, as a vegetarian who eats loads of green vegetables I wouldn't have developed breast cancer at thirty-three. All the doctors I've seen have said you should eat whatever you want.

- Don't be taken in by alternative treatments. Chemotherapy and radiotherapy and surgery will give you the best chance. If you go down the natural route, you're not giving yourself the best chance.

- Nature and animals. Dog-walking has really helped me – I find dogs so calming to be with and I love being out walking with them. If you have a pet, make sure to spend time with them, and if you don't have one think about joining Borrow My Doggy so you can walk someone else's dog or spend time with them in their or your home. This is how I met Mr Fluffypants and he helped me so much – he changed my life. Also, gardening probably helps if you do that, or visiting gardens and wild places. I'm a member of London and Whipsnade Zoos and visit regularly – they're my happy places and it always cheers me up to see the animals.

- You're stronger than you think. There were some things that terrified me – chemotherapy, the thought of losing my hair, surgery. I dreaded these things and then they happened, and I coped with them. The ability of the human spirit to survive is remarkable.

- Social media. When I've been bed-bound or confined to my parents' house, just connecting with other people through Facebook and Instagram and Wordpress has really helped me feel less alone. I joined a worldwide Facebook group for young women with breast cancer and I've learnt some useful things there – I got the idea to ask for bisphosphonates, which help to protect bones against cancer, from an American friend in the group who was taking them.

- Creative pastimes: Blogging and writing, drawing, making collages and knitting have really helped me. At the beginning, when I'd just been diagnosed with breast cancer, I had art therapy. It wasn't brilliant for me but could be for someone who didn't get so frustrated about their drawing having deteriorated over the years. Knitting has been a lifesaver – it's portable, doesn't make a mess, you have to concentrate on it and yet can do it in front of the television, it keeps your hands busy and eventually you will have something to wear or to give to someone as a present.

What Not to Say to Someone with A Life-Threatening Illness

- "You've got to keep fighting." No, they haven't. This is neither a war, nor a boxing match. Chances are, if you're having chemotherapy or radiotherapy, you'll be exhausted, vomiting, sleeping, collapsed on the sofa. You won't be clad in armour and swinging a mace around.

- "You've got to be positive." Recent studies have shown a positive attitude has no effect whatsoever on outcomes. You haven't got to be anything, and it's no one's business how you feel about having suddenly acquired a life-threatening illness. Be however you want. Of course, if you can, keep up as many as possible of your normal activities as it might help you feel better. If it makes you feel better to spend your months of treatment in bed or watching *Poirot* on the sofa eight hours a day, that's fine too.

- "You're so strong, you'll beat this illness." Physical or mental strength may have an impact on how quickly your body recovers from the after-effects of certain treatments, or they may not. At chemotherapy, a lot of the septuagenarians were laughing and joking with each other as they sat up in chairs hooked up to their drips. Some patients even wheeled their drips outside so they could have a fag every forty minutes. On the other hand, I lay collapsed in bed, dozing, despite my age (thirty-four) and my five gym sessions per week. Despite exercising all the way through my treatment, I spent the five weeks of radiotherapy asleep or collapsed in front of *Poirot* or *Marple* on the sofa. My apparent youth and strength made no difference whatsoever.

- "Everything will be fine after the operation." This one was and still is a major source of irritation to me, my parents and my brother. The cancer was in my skin, there weren't going to be clear margins, the operation was going to be an eight-hour epic where the hump I'd been growing on my back was flipped over to my front. All my lymph nodes were coming out, there was a huge risk of lymphoedema, an enormous section of back muscle would be carved out and a whole boob lopped off. There would be months of recuperation. Everything would not be fine after the operation.

- Blanket statements such as, "I know you'll get through this / overcome this / you're stronger than this / you'll get better." No, you don't know anything of the kind. We hope I won't die of it, so please say that instead.

- Minimising language, "I hear you're a bit poorly" and suchlike. I'm not a bit poorly! I've got a terminal illness. By and large the reactions we found helpful and supportive have been people saying, "Oh my G-d, how awful, poor you, I can't imagine what you must be going through," or a kind cousin who said, "I can't imagine how I would feel if this was one of my daughters" or "You're too young for this" or "You've been through so much already". Don't be afraid to say how awful or unfair you think it is that your friend or relative has been diagnosed with this horrible illness. A genuine expression of horror will be far more appreciated than an attempt to minimise the suffering of the ill person.

- It's fine not to talk about the illness or treatment but simply to do something nice for your friend or relative. When I'd just received my cancer diagnosis and started chemo, a friend arranged for us to get Minx foil wraps on our toenails (brilliant – they last for about six weeks). That was a lovely gesture and really appreciated.

- Don't make offers of help such as "I'll take you to chemo" unless you really intend to do it. Likewise, "If there's anything I can do to help, just ask" is not helpful as the ill person or their family just won't ask. What we really hoped people would offer to do were simple practical things: taking me to the supermarket when I was trying to manage in the flat alone between chemo and the operation, for example. Usually, we didn't feel like going out for dinner for hours or to the theatre, and after about twenty minutes we'd had enough of visitors. Mum hated it when people phoned every day to ask, "How are you?" She didn't want to talk on the phone, and after all, there was nothing to say.

- "Have you tried eating broccoli / cutting out dairy / drinking spirulina? My friend had prostate cancer and he cured it by injecting himself with satay sauce / snorting lentils / kale suppositories." Please don't share your quack remedies or diet myths. The ill person is being poisoned by chemotherapy and burnt by radiotherapy. They would rather not be having these horrible treatments, but by and large they have the most successful outcomes. It is amusing when people start with "Have you tried broccoli?" I'm vegetarian and eat a couple of heads of broccoli per day. My poo is green. If broccoli had a protective effect against cancer, I wouldn't have got it in the first place.

- Please try and think before expressing an opinion about the ill person's chances, prognosis, treatment or any of the above. Or before asking, "So what did your oncologist say?" Chances are the ill person can't remember what their oncologist said or spent their appointment crying and telling them "I hate you". And the patient doesn't want to give a blow-by-blow account of every appointment to everyone who asks. It's just none of your business. We found it helpful for Dad to send a group email out to friends and family explaining what was happening after certain crucial appointments or operations. Some people set up a Facebook group and page for their illness and post updates there.

- Another pet hate, particularly of Mum's, is people who, on hearing of my diagnosis, said, "Oh my grandma got breast cancer when she was seventy, she recovered and died of something else years later" and then launch into an exhaustive account of their grandma's treatment aged seventy-three for a different form of breast cancer in the early 1970s. The people who featured in these anecdotes were all far older than me, with far less extensive tumours, so their experience was irrelevant. These stories are of very limited use anyway: everyone's cancer behaves in a different way.

- "Wow you're on such a journey. You're going to learn so much." The concept of the "Cancer journey", as peddled by women's magazines, is another thing that annoys us. The prevalence of the notion that cancer would act on the successful businesswoman's life as a wake-up call, encouraging her to cut down her working hours to spend more time with her husband and children just didn't apply to me. Aged thirty-three, stuck in an entry-level job, single, diagnosed bipolar 1 aged twenty-four, the last thing I needed was to slow down, smell the flowers and so on and so on. I'd done all that years ago, in recovery from my mental disorder. I object to the whole idea of the "Cancer journey" anyway, and all that "What doesn't kill you makes you stronger" stuff.

This last one stems, I think, from people's fear and horror of severe illness. They shrink away from the unpleasant physical realities of the treatments and such side effects as hair loss, surgery, drains and even blood. The calmest people were my cat's vets, the ladies at carriage driving, country friends who experience the cycle of life and death on farms and Mum's science teacher friends.

My parental friends are, perhaps inevitably, better at dealing with me than my younger friends when I am undergoing treatment. Some of my cousins are brilliant. My boss, tragically now dead from breast cancer herself, was wonderful, sending little presents and cards all the time. Don't underestimate the power of a handwritten card – it was, and is, so good to receive them.

Some gestures stand out years later: my mum's biology teacher colleague who turned up with an orange drizzle cake as soon as she heard; my boss arranging tickets for my best friend Hannah and me to see *American Psycho* at the Almeida; being taken by my uncle to see Watford play at Wembley (we wuz robbed); and the gift of the world's best kitten from my much-loved ex-boyfriend Seb. My next-door neighbour at the flat also watered my plants whilst I was in hospital, which was a great help.

I wish there was a list of ten things *to* say. Maybe next time. The main thing is to be genuine, be over-dramatic rather than minimising, or simply turn up armed with a hug, a smile and a little treat.

Chapter 26

NOVEMBER 2016

I'm out with Mr Fluffypants the Keeshond in Belsize Park. We approach a bench. We've been walking for a while. Sitting down, I notice a young man next to me. He's wearing Chelsea boots, tight black jeans and a leather jacket and has shoulder-length light brown hair.

"Hi," I say, gripped by a sudden impulse to speak to him.

"Hi," he says, looking at me with clear blue eyes. He has delicate features, he's pretty rather than handsome but there's something about him.

"What are you up to?" I ask.

"Oh, I'm looking at properties in the area," he says. "I'm looking to move here and ..."

"Where are you from?" I ask.

"Australia originally but I've been at music college up North – I'm a musician, a guitarist, so ..."

"That's great," I say. "I live round here. So does the pooch – he's not mine, I walk him for some people, but give me a call if you move here and I'll show you around."

"Great. What's your number?" he asks, taking his phone out of his pocket.

Telling him my number, watching him write it into his phone, I smile at him. "Look forward to hearing from you," I say.

"Sure," he says, smiling at me.

"Come on, Mr Fluffypants," I say, standing up, starting the walk back to his flat.

"Hi, it's Josh. We met in Belsize Park," the message comes through a few days later. "I've moved to Camden. Wondering if you want to meet?"

"Sure. Great to hear from you. Come round for dinner on Saturday," I reply.

This is exciting, I think. *A cute young chap wants to see me.*

Saturday arrives. I put some make-up and a dress on, put some pizzas in the oven and make a salad. *This is exciting to be at the flat at the weekend, waiting for a chap*, I think.

The entry phone buzzes, and I let him in. He's wearing his leather jacket again and his hair is shoulder-length, mid-brown. He wears tight black jeans, black Chelsea boots and a black sweater.

"Would you like a Diet Coke," I ask. "I gave up drinking and …"

"Sure," he says.

We sit on my bed and drink our Diet Cokes.

"Do you like Leonard Cohen?" I ask.

"Yes, of course," he says.

I put on *The Future*.

"So, tell me," I say, looking at him. "What are you doing in London?"

He pushes a lock of hair behind his ear. "So, I'm a musician, I've got a single coming out and …"

"How old are you?"

"Twenty-three," he says.

Gosh, that is young, I think. It's cheering that someone so young likes Leonard Cohen. It's good, of course, to have attracted his attention but I'm thirty-seven and … *there's no point in worrying about this now*, I decide.

"I'm a bit older than you," I say.

"That's OK," he says.

"So, what sort of music do you do?" I ask.

"Oh, you know, singer-songwriter stuff," he says. "I play the guitar – I teach the guitar too …"

"That's great," I say.

I seem to have acquired a boyfriend. We have a wonderful time and I have another date arranged with Josh for the following Saturday. This is exciting and unexpected. I haven't been with anyone since I split up with Seb back in March and it's now November. So, it's fabulous to have an evening with my new boy to look forward to. It's exciting to have someone to think about – this slim indie boy who's not my usual sort of thing at all. He's impressive though, at twenty-three to be earning enough from being a session musician and teaching guitar to be able to afford to move to Camden. *Things are looking up*, I think.

Saturday night and I'm waiting for Josh again.

"I like peculiar people, you're peculiar," he says as we sit in my room listening to *Songs of Leonard Cohen*.

"Thank you," I say realising that it's meant to be a compliment.

"I'm playing a gig in February – would you like to come?" he asks.

"Yes, I'd love that," I say.

"It's at the Half Moon in Putney," he says.

"I've never been there," I say.

"It's a cool venue, I've played there before," he says.

"I'll definitely come," I say, thinking I can ask my cousin Patrick who lives near there to come.

The next day, I go to the website for the venue and buy two tickets. I message my friend Becky to see if she'll come with me and she replies to say she'll sort out a babysitter and she'll come. So that's good. *It will be so exciting to see my boy singing and playing the guitar,*

I think. It's taken me till the age of thirty-seven to get a boyfriend in a band, but better late than never. It's great to have something to look forward to. I thought I'd never meet anyone after Seb and yet here I am, with a new twenty-three-year-old boyfriend. *It just goes to show*, I think, *you never know what's just around the corner*.

I'm sitting in Dr Stein's office.

"Dr Stein," I say. "I think I've got PTSD."

"Why is that?" he asks, looking concerned.

"Well, I'm still really upset about Seb splitting up with me," I say. "And he split up with me when I was at my flat and so I don't like being there, and every time I'm there I think about it, and it's not getting better, it's getting worse, I have these horrible flashbacks and …"

"That isn't what I'd expect," Dr Stein says, scribbling in my notes. "Your memory of Seb splitting up with you should be fading by now, it certainly shouldn't be getting worse. Now, what you need for PTSD is a treatment called EMDR – Eye Movement Deregulation Therapy – I know a psychologist who does it. Would you like me to write to her to see if she has space for you?"

"Yes, please," I say. "That would be great."

"OK, I'll email her and she'll be in touch with you. See you in a couple of weeks," he says.

"Thank you, Dr Stein," I say.

"Take care," he says, giving me a hug as I head out of the door.

Just after Christmas and I'm house-sitting with Mary. We go to her friend Cynthia's house which is just down the road: a pretty cottage next to a farm where a bronze turkey clucks at us as we walk past him.

"Cynthia's going to teach you to knit," Mary says. Sitting on a sofa, under a furry throw, I ask "where's Diego?" Diego is Cynthia's cat – he's a Ragamuffin: a bit like Spitfire but silver with a huge fluffy tail – Mary calls him 'the snow leopard'.

"He's just outside," Cynthia says. She sits on a sofa under another furry blanket. The fire burns in the grate. It's a warm, comfortable room. "I'm going to cast on a row for you and then I'm going to let you take over because casting on is difficult."

"Thank you," I say.

She casts on a row of stitches. "These needles are good," she says. "They're wooden so they feel nice. Now you take over."

"What do I do?" I ask, holding the needle with the one row of stitches in my hand.

"Slide the other needle in, then wind the wool round it, then push the needle under and take the stitch off the first needle onto the second needle, that's right," Cynthia says, guiding my hand. "Now just repeat 'til the end of the row – I've only cast on twenty stitches for you …"

"I've brought you here to see Cynthia because I'm not sure how to teach someone to knit," Mary says, from under another furry blanket where she's getting on with her own knitting project.

Pushing the right needle under the left, I twist a piece of wool from the right to divide the stitch, push my right needle under the left, lifting the stitch onto the right needle. I repeat this until I reach the end of the row.

"Very good," Cynthia says. "Make sure not to pull the wool too tight or you'll make it difficult for yourself."

"OK," I say, starting the second row. Push needle, wind wool, lift stitch to other needle, repeat. Push needle, wind wool, lift stitch to other needle, repeat.

"I thought we could go to the wool shop in town tomorrow," Mary says.

"Oh yes, I've wanted to go there for ages," Cynthia says.

"I'd love that," I say. "I can get some yarn and make something and …"

"I'll pick you up tomorrow afternoon," Cynthia says. "Oh look, here he is. Hello Diego."

The majestic cat stalks over to where we're sitting.

"Please may I take a photo of him?" I ask. "So I can show my Mum?"

"Of course you can," Cynthia says. The cat sits down, magnificent tail wrapped around his paws. Snapping a few shots, I think I've captured him.

"We'd better get going," Mary says.

"Do you want to take the needles and the wool and give them back to me tomorrow?" Cynthia asks me.

"Thank you, that's so kind of you," I say.

"Make sure not to sit on them – they're wood so they'll break," she says.

We're at the knitting shop. It's amazing: one side of the shop is shelves of acrylic yarn and that's the one I want because I'm allergic to wool. I find some brightly coloured yarn called Cabaret Sunset which is fuchsia pink, purple, blue, orange and mustard with a bright blue lurex thread going through it. Picking up a few balls, I find the same needles Cynthia has lent me in the shop and go to pay for all of it.

"I want everything," Mary says, picking up a ball of thick green wool with different colours in it from the reduced-to-clear basket.

"I think this would be nice for a scarf," Cynthia says, picking up a ball of scarlet wool with black sequins threaded into it. "I'm going to get a few balls of this."

We head back to the car, past the church. It's getting dark already.

"Why don't you come back and do some knitting with us?" Mary says to Cynthia.

"Oh, alright then," Cynthia says. "That will be fun."

"Cynthia, would you please cast on some stitches for me when we get back?" I ask, holding my bag of precious wool and needles.

"Of course I will," she says.

Back at the house, Tammi, the elderly chocolate Labrador we're looking after, sits next to Mary on one sofa and I sit next to Cynthia on the other one. The sofas are at right angles to each other.

"So how many stitches would you like me to cast on for you?" Cynthia asks.

"I'd like it to be about as wide as the scarf I've been wearing," I say, going into the hall and bringing my scarf over to show her. "This one."

"I'd say about sixty stitches then," Cynthia says, examining my infinity scarf. "Right, I'll cast on sixty stitches for you – you carry on with that little square for the moment."

"OK," I say, getting back to work on my little green square.

Mary is stroking Tammi's tummy. The elderly Labrador stretches out, content.

This is a happy knitting scene. I can't believe I can knit and I'm going to be working on a scarf.

"Thank you so much, both of you, for teaching me to knit and taking me to the wool shop," I say.

"I've been meaning to go there for ages, just hadn't got round to it," Cynthia says, casting on stitches.

"It's lovely there," Mary says, knitting with the green wool she's just bought.

"I'm having such a nice time," I say. I do feel better to be out of London, seeing my best friend, getting away from the soul-crushing tedium of my routine and doing something else. And now I can knit I'll be able to amuse myself for the rest of the winter.

"The thing about knitting," Mary says, "is that it's not messy like other crafts. It's portable and you can just put it down in a ball. There isn't any clearing up to do."

"You should get a knitting bag," Cynthia says. "So you can take it out with you. Do you want me to cast off that green square so you can keep it as a memento of your first bit of knitting?"

"Oh yes please," I say.

"Then I can have my needles back as you've got your own needles now," she says.

"I'm just going to make us some supper," Mary says, going through to the kitchen.

"There you go," Cynthia says, handing me the little green square. "Your first piece of knitting."

"Thank you," I say, turning it over with wonder. It's a little square, about five centimetres by five centimetres, but it's my first knitted item. "I love it." I say.

Chapter 27

JANUARY 2017

"How was your trip?" Alicia asks. She's my new psychologist. We're sitting in the treatment room: I'm on one big sofa sitting with my feet tucked under me, knitting. She's sitting in an armchair next to me.

"Good, I think," I say. "Let me just count the stitches – I've reached the end of a row." I count to sixty under my breath. "Yes, I had a good trip. Mary's friend Cynthia taught me to knit."

"So I see," Alicia says. "Have you been doing a lot of it?"

"Yes, all the time." I say. "In front of the television and when I'm in bed listening to music."

"That's good to hear," Alicia says. I really like her a lot. She's about my age: tall and blonde – she's half-Norwegian – and very bright. I find her easy to talk to. "So how are you feeling about Seb?"

"Well, I still miss him," I say. "But it's not as bad as it was. I've met this new man and he takes my mind off Seb a bit – I'm going to his gig next month – he's a musician."

"That's great," Alicia says. "Where did you meet him?"

"Belsize Park. When I was walking Mr Fluffypants," I say, knitting. "He's twenty-three but he's grown up for his age – he earns enough money teaching the guitar and being a session musician to rent in Camden."

"Impressive," she says.

We haven't started the EMDR yet. We've decided to get to know each other first. It makes a difference to me to have someone to talk to for fifty minutes per week about what's going on in my life. And I really like Alicia. I feel less alone now.

"Do you want to talk about Seb?" Alicia asks.

I shake my head. "Not really, not now. I'm trying to move on."

"Are you still feeling the same about being in your flat?" Alicia asks. "Do you still not want to be there because that's where he split up with you?"

"No," I say. "It feels OK being there."

"It sounds like time is healing. It does that," she says.

"I didn't think it would," I say. "I thought my heart would be broken forever."

"Well, that tends not to be what happens – you do start to heal from a broken heart," she says. And none of this is that profound, but it's true. I am feeling better. I know Seb isn't coming back and I'm coming to terms with that and getting on with my life – at least with the part of my life that includes dating a new boy.

"I didn't think it would happen," I say. "I thought my heart would be broken forever – I mean there are times, like when the Brexit vote happened last summer I really wanted to talk to him about it, but a lot of the time I'm OK."

"That's good," Alicia says. "You're moving on. The memories are fading."

"I wrote a poem about the new boy, and knitting, do you want to hear it?" I ask.

"Yeah, sure, why not?"

"It's called 'I Wind My Wool Around Your Heart'," I say. Clearing my throat, I find the poem on my phone, and start to read:

"When you leave it's needle sharp.
I knit this blanket round your soul –
Just feel the softness of the yarn.
You say you want to be alone –
I answer: knit one purl one.
You say this isn't what you want.
I turn the needles, start another row.
There are more things in heaven and earth
Than can be solved by balling wool –
And for the rest there's sleep and tea.
Don't disappoint me when you leave –
I know this isn't forever, darling:
But stay with me for now.
I knit our love into a scarf
To wrap around your neck at night
To hold you tight between
The stitches of my pain
Drop one, pick it up again.
Even more now than before
I know you'll leave and pull this thread,
Unravelling my work as I cry in bed –
Helpless to halt the unpicking of this place
Where all I want's your heart, your face.
Your hair curls across my pillow
Where we are happy, and together weave
A blanket of all our shared dreams.
The lurex thread that runs through my yarn
I wind it through your silken hair
Breathe into your ear again
"You are mine and we must rest"
You lie back upon my bed

Sink into the memory foam.
You are the centre of my world
The scarf of our love unfurled.
I wrap my wool around your soul
To bind us tight against the endless night."

"That's beautiful," Alicia says.

"Do you like it?" I say.

"I like it so much," she says. "I think it's great that you're writing poetry."

"It's the young songwriter boy," I say. "He inspires me to do something with my own talents."

"That's wonderful," she says, smiling at me. "So, I'll see you next week, same time?"

"Ten o'clock next Wednesday," I say, pushing my needles into the ball of wool, winding the knitting round them, putting it in my knitting bag. Unplugging my phone from the charger on the wall, pulling my boots on, I take my coat down from the hook on the door.

"Bye," I say, picking up all my stuff.

"See you next week, take care," Alicia says, smiling at me.

Stepping out onto the street, it's a bright sunny day. Feeling cheerful, I put the *ABBA Gold* playlist on my phone, put my earphones in, and start the thirty-minute walk back to my flat along the main road.

Chapter 28

"What are you drinking," I ask my friend Becky as we stand at the bar at the Half Moon in Putney

"Rum and Coke please," she says. I order that for Becky and a Diet Coke with fresh lime for me: I'm still not drinking, of course. We're waiting for my cousin Patrick, to see Josh in concert. I'm excited. I'm wearing a short purple dress printed with the universe – the same print as on the cover of Josh's single.

The bar is long and mirrored – this is probably a Victorian pub, I reckon. It's south of the river. Becky lives near here in Richmond.

Sitting at our table with our drinks, we chat and wait for Patrick who's coming after a job interview. It feels good, if a bit strange, to be out at night, preparing to watch a concert. I can't remember the last time I went out at night to a gig. Finally, for the first time in my life, I'm dating a musician.

"I'm excited to see your chap on stage," Becky says.

"He should be good," I say. "The single is brilliant – did I send it to you?"

"Yes, you did," she says. "So, I'm using a new babysitter tonight –now I'm young, free and single I'd like to get out a bit more." Becky is a widow.

"I should get out more," I say. "It's difficult now I'm not drinking though – I just want to stay in in the evening and listen to Leonard Cohen and knit."

"Well, you're out now," she says. "Which is great. You saw Mary, didn't you?" We all met on the old Manic Depression Fellowship internet forum fourteen years ago. How time flies.

"Yeah, I was house-sitting with her over New Year," I say, sipping my Diet Coke.

"How was she?" Becky asks.

"She was good," I say. "Her friend Cynthia taught me to knit, and I rode one of the horses, which was lovely."

"Hello girls," my cousin Patrick says, arriving at our table wearing a suit and looking very smart. He's six foot three – his dad's family are very tall – with film star looks. I lived with him for two weeks some years ago now and remember him walking around dressed in a towel: so gorgeous even though, of course, he's my cousin.

"Hi Patrick," I say. "This is Becky, she's one of my bipolar lot."

"Pleased to meet you, Becky," Patrick says, extending a hand to shake hers. I watch for Becky's reaction to my gorgeous cousin. She bats her lashes at him. "What are you drinking?"

"Diet Coke, please," I say.

"Rum and Coke please," Becky says.

"I just left the office and I realised this place was on my way home," Patrick says, returning to the table with the drinks. "And I thought I'd drop by and have a look at this boy."

"I hope he's good," I say. "The single is brilliant. Can't wait to see him perform live."

There's a commotion behind the bar as the doors to the band room open.

We pay at the door and walk into the room, standing near the stage. The band are setting up. I see Josh and smile at him.

"He's that one," I say to Becky and Patrick.

"He's not your usual sort of thing," Becky, sounding surprised. I tend to go for tall, well-built men.

"No, I know," I say, watching my skinny indie boyfriend tuning his guitar.

"So, this song is called 'Ilona' and it's about an old girlfriend, who's actually here with her new boyfriend so I'm not sure how I feel about that," Josh says, launching into a song.

He looks really hot up there singing and playing his guitar, his long hair falling over his face. He's wearing tight black skinny jeans and a black shirt with white flowers on, with the top couple of buttons undone. It's dark and we're dancing. I'm having fun, I realise. I can't remember the last time I went out at night and danced.

"So now we're going to play the new single," Josh says. "It's called 'Talk To G-d.' I hope you like it."

The single is a belter.

"Really good," Becky says, clapping with her hands above her head, dancing. I'm so glad she's having fun – she's had a rough year since her husband's sudden death from lung cancer.

He's wonderful, I think. *Well done me to have landed such a talented young boyfriend.*

Patrick walks off at some point and I hang around with Becky till the end of the concert. The lights come up. Josh disappears behind the stage.

"Is it OK if we just wait for him to come out?" I ask, feeling very tired all of a sudden. It's late, I'm far from home – the cab here cost me thirty pounds.

"Yeah, sure, but then I've got to get going," Becky says.

I want to congratulate Josh on his performance.

At long last he comes out. "Thank you for coming," he says, but he seems distracted as he kisses me on the cheek. "There are some people here I have to talk to," he says.

"It was great. You were wonderful," I say.

"Glad you could make it," he says, wandering off.

"I guess we can go now," I say to Becky, feeling a sense of anticlimax. *Josh didn't seem particularly pleased to see me*, I think, as I say goodbye to my friend and order an Uber. I thought he might come back to the flat with me, or at least want to have a drink together at the end of the gig.

Waking up the next morning, I send Josh a message. "Wonderful performance last night, you were brilliant." No reply. I'm tired after a late night but I drag myself to the gym to lift some weights, feeling unsettled. *He didn't behave last night as if he was pleased to see me*, I think as I sit on the leg press, lifting 140kg. He didn't behave like he was my boyfriend.

"Hi," the message comes through from Josh, at last, sometime in the afternoon. "I think we want really different things out of this relationship so I don't think we should see each other anymore."

I knew this was coming, I tell myself, as the tears start rolling down my cheeks. It was obvious from his behaviour last night. But it's still a shock, and it's a shame. I've enjoyed spending time with him. It's been good having someone else to think about after the whole Seb business. I suppose it was inevitable, what with him being twenty-three. *It's not my fault*, I tell myself.

"OK," I reply. Then I delete him from my Facebook and unfollow his band page. The signed poster from his gig sits on my bookshelf, rolled up and fastened with an elastic band. *I won't be getting that one framed*, I tell myself, as I retire to bed with my Leonard Cohen box set and my knitting.

And just like that, I'm single again. I've spent most of my life being single after all. When I was at university there was my first boyfriend, Jeremy, for twenty months and then more recently there was Seb – for five months when I was twenty-six, then again for four months when I was thirty before he entered the monastery, and then our last go at the relationship when I was thirty-six, for thirteen months. But apart from that, I've been single most of my life, with occasional short relationships punctuating the desert.

When you're often single, you acclimatise to things: enjoying a film alone, having no plus one at weddings. You get accustomed to doing things your own way and to not having a partner at family events; to having no one to snuggle and watch television with over the long winter months.

So, Josh is gone and I'm back to my natural single state. Unfortunately, this period coincides with a long stretch of time where I'm at loggerheads with my best friend, Lily. The problems started when she had a baby eighteen months ago and we just haven't really been able to maintain our friendship since then.

"I suppose I feel," I say to Alicia. "When Lily needed me, when her brother was dying, I was a brilliant friend to her. And now I need her ... well, since I've had my breast cancer diagnosis she's married and had a baby and she just hasn't been there for me so ..."

"And how does that make you feel?" Alicia asks.

"Disappointed," I say. "Disappointed in her. And now I just don't want to spend time with her, which I know isn't helping. I don't want to lose the friendship and yet I also don't want to sort things out with her because I feel so irritated with her: it's difficult. Hang on a second, I need to count this row," I say, counting sixty stitches.

"So, what do you think would help?" Alicia asks.

"Well, she's sent me a few dates to meet, and I suppose I'll have to see her on one of them but I just don't want to," I say.

"If she's given you some dates to meet, why not pick one a bit further away." Alicia says." And maybe you'll feel more like seeing her when the time comes or ..."

"OK, that sounds sensible," I say. "I've written another poem, about weightlifting. Would you like to hear it?"

"Yes, sure," Alicia says, smiling at me.

"It's called 'Clean and Jerk'," I say, "Which is a move in weightlifting:

I lift to fill the cavern of my heart
Where you have been and yet won't stay.
I lift to grasp the fleet-footed day
Who won't be held, who sprints away.
I lift to strengthen my weakened bones,
Which cancer drugs aim to leach away.
I lift to grasp the charging bull by his horns.
I lift: urging him to turn another way.
I lift to fill my empty soul,
Where dogs drop in then trot away.
Leaving nothing but wisps of fur
To show they've even been here at all.
I lift to expand the weak winter sun,
To pull him from the clouds wherein he stays.
I lift because there's nothing else that helps,
When days are dark and nights too long.
I lift because I cannot write a song.
Because the words they always flit away –
Just out of reach of all my new intent
To frame my world so it makes sense.
I lift, bolstering my shaking confidence,
To build on the small progress I have made
With bars and bells and weighted balls:
I need to up my targets of them all.
And in the spaces between

What I need and what I own
I lift because we are all alone.
Alone on this darkening plain
Of fear and endless blame.
The forests shrink, the seas recede,
The fires burn, a desperate need
For comfort and freedom from fear,
Which can't be calmed
Except by lifting weights.
And is it luck or is it fate
Or is it something else instead.
Without the chink of light
We'll all be dead.
And as the reaper rides
Towards me at a canter,
I know that lifting
Weights must be the answer.
Behind the clouds
The winter sun breaks through:
My body aches
And yet my spirit's resolute.
To rise and meet
The challenges of pain –
I start another set
Of tricep lifts, again.
And on and on
Through winter fog and sleet,
After lifting I know
That I will sleep
And dream of sunlit uplands,
Leaping lambs

Of lynx in forests,
Beavers building dams.
Wolves will return and
With them a kind of hope,
That maybe the whole world
Just might not implode.
A slim hope, and
Yet worth writing here.
I lift to dull the
Constant ache of fear
And age, and decline
And mental anguish.
For all of this,
I speak the simple language
Of lift then rest
Then lift then rest again
Till what comes is
The long-foretold end
Of love and life and hope
And all those things.
Lifting centres me
Within the silent scream."

"That's great," Alicia says. "I'm glad you're writing all this poetry. So, I'll see you at the same time next week?"

"See you then," I say, collecting my knitting and all my bags and getting to my feet.

"Come on, Dolly," I say. I'm out with my new dog client, a black Newfoundland. I met her and her owner when I was out with Hannah walking Mr Fluffypants and now I pick her up every

Tuesday in Belsize Park. We're walking up Primrose Hill and Dolly is dawdling as she's wont to do, what with being a giant.

It's a crisp February day and I'm wearing a coat, gloves and grey furry infinity scarf. The cold is bracing as we trek up the hill. It's a big effort with this huge lumbering beast beside me. Dolly is two and still thinks she's a baby: when I arrive at her house she likes to rugby tackle me from behind. I'm meant to stand up straight with my back to her, cross my arms and say "No" in a loud voice until she gets down. She still does it every week though – she's still an excitable young puppy at heart.

We arrive at the top of the hill. "Excuse me," I say to a girl sitting on a bench, "do you mind taking a photo of us please?"

Dolly has gone up to her and put her head in the girl's lap. She's such a sweet, gentle giant.

"Sure," the girl says, stroking the big furry head. "Your dog is gorgeous. What sort of dog is she?"

"She's a Newfoundland," I say. "She's just a big baby really. Come on Dolly," I say, leading her over to sit next to me on the little ledge at the top of the hill. Behind us you can see the whole of London stretching away into the distance. Putting my arm round my furry chum, I look at the camera.

"OK, I've taken a few," the girl says. "Do you want to have a look?" She hands me my camera. I can see a couple of good shots. Dolly's head is about twice the size of mine – she's such a big girl.

"Thank you very much," I say. "Come on Dolly."

We amble down the hill, turn left at the bottom and we're soon out of the park. We walk through Primrose Hill, past Lemonia, the Greek restaurant on our left and a couple of flower shops, the Pamela Shiffer designer clothes shop, Nicolas wines, the Cowshed Spa and the Mary Portas Living & Giving charity shop. We cross the bridge – Fierce Grace yoga on our right and a coffee shop on our left – and head towards Chalk Farm station. At the station we turn left up Rosslyn Hill to head back to Belsize Park and have a rest outside the church. I sit on a bench, give Dolly a treat and take a couple of photos of her.

As I arise from the bench, Dolly heaves herself to her feet and pads along besides me on huge paws. I pass The Load of Hay on our right – the pub where I spent that evening with Seb and his sister Katie. This area is rich in memories of Seb: the Sir Richard Steele pub is on our left, where we went on the day he dumped me. We take a left into England's Lane, walking past the old-fashioned pharmacy on our right and the Winchester pub. This is one of my favourite walks – I'm always calm and settled when I'm out with Dolly. The padding of her big paws on the pavement soothes my anxiety.

Turning right into Dolly's road, we pass big white Georgian houses on both sides of the road. Ringing the bell, I hear Dolly's owner come to the door.

"Was she a good girl?" Dolly's owner, Nina, asks me. She's a slight woman in her mid-seventies who's an old hippie: there are CND signs and Green Party posters up in the hall.

"She was such a good girl," I say, handing Dolly over.

"Oh good," Nina says, smiling at the giant girl and stroking the soft top of her head. Dolly lies down, taking up most of the room.

"Thank you very much," Nina says, handing me a ten-pound note.

"No, thank you for letting me walk her," I say, putting the money in my purse. "I love her."

"Well, she's ever so fond of you," Nina says.

"Goodbye Dolly, see you next week," I say, stroking the soft back of her neck.

"Thank you," Nina calls after me. Pulling the door to behind me, I walk back to the station to catch the train home.

Chapter 29

SUMMER 2016

"No, you've got to get the plastic box over the top of her," Mum says. A wren is trapped in the house, in the living room, at the back under the sloping windows. We're trying to catch her but it's impossible. The miniscule brown bird evades our attempts to pin her against the window with the Tupperware box: flapping her wings, jumping, flying out of our reach.

"I'm trying my best," I say to Mum. The wren hops free, behind the radiator, and I can't get the box near her.

"We're not going to be able to go on holiday," says, Mum looking worried. We are about to set off to visit Mum's best friend in her second home in the Dordogne. Heart hammering in my chest, I move the plastic box towards the bird, but she hops away, taking up residence behind the radiator. Sliding the box towards her again, she answers by beating her wings, flying up the window towards the ceiling. We're frozen in fear.

The wren of anxiety flies down my throat and into my stomach and zooms around, her wings beating. She flaps around my stomach and I'm rooted to the spot, paralysed.

This is anxiety. I probably should put this much earlier in the book because I experience this in both phases of my illness, when my mood is high or low. It's one of the reasons why I find it so difficult to get out of the house in the morning. I'll wake up and have breakfast at eight o'clock but the anxiety wren flies around my stomach, rooting me to the spot until sometimes eleven o'clock. That's three hours of being unable to break free and press on with my day.

Once I'm outside, I just know everyone's looking at me, that people are talking about me. The wren flutters around my stomach, her wings beating in my head. The weight of the sky presses down on me with ominous intent. Something terrible is about to happen. Just what it is remains vague, but no less severe for that.

When I stop drinking, the wren takes up residence in my stomach. I take clonazepam to help with the anxiety but sometimes it's not enough. I used to venture out at night in search of drink but now the wren keeps me at home. I'm attending the cinema at 5.30 p.m. this afternoon just to force myself out of the house. I'll take a cab to and from the cinema, but I'll be out, around other people and I know that's good for me. The best way to fight the anxiety can be to confront it by doing something low-key.

There's an extra layer of anxiety now I'm not drinking. The alcohol itself used to quieten the beating of the wren's wings, lulling me into feeling better, at least for the evening. Now if I go to a party I feel exposed and don't know what to do with myself. I hover by the food or find a pet to talk to. I'll become acclimatised to it in the end but I think it's still at too early a stage in my recovery from alcoholism to attend parties. I'm missing the Spin Christmas Party because it's a gin and tonic evening and that was my tipple of choice. Sad, but there it is. I have to look after myself.

When I was really thin and looked great, I had to attend a pool party where I decided to wear a bikini. I've never felt comfortable in a bikini and this was in Houston. *Everyone will be thinner than me and tanned*, I remember thinking. My mood was at rock bottom at that time – it was at the tail end of our "trip of a lifetime" holiday to Canada where I'd been so depressed the whole time. Looking back on the photos, I look amazing. But mental illness doesn't care about such things. So, I put on my bikini, dipped into the pool, hauled myself out again and dressed as fast as possible.

How I Combat Anxiety

- Reduce caffeine which feeds it.
- Meditate: this has been proven to help sufferers and I find doing the 20 minute body scan before bed helps me sleep. I also do it before my afternoon sleep. Put "20 minute body scan" into Google and that will bring up the Palouse Mindfulness page which has the body scan I use. You can download it onto your phone.
- Venture outside in the fresh air. Know that this is easier said than done but it helps.
- Walk: see above. Walking is a form of meditation in itself and being in nature, listening to birdsong and looking at trees can help.
- Avoid crowded places. The London Underground has just published a new map of which stations are above ground for people who are anxious or claustrophobic and want to avoid tunnels.
- Learn how to breathe in a mindful, calming way. Diaphragmatic breathing – which we do in Pilates – is the best.
- Spend time with pets. Stroking a dog or cat has been proven to reduce anxiety.
- If no pets are on offer, visit the zoo – this always helps me – or a local farm or just watch the birds in your garden.
- If your anxiety is really bad, please see a medical professional. You may need Cognitive Behaviour Therapy or drugs.

- See friends. This can help a lot.
- Exercise. I never feel anxious when my mind and body are occupied lifting weights, or at Pilates, or barre, or swimming in a pool or best of all in the sea.
- There are no magic answers. Sometimes you will only be able to lie under a blanket watching television, but that's fine.
- Knitting: gives you something to do with your hands and you have to concentrate on counting the stitches at the end of each row. Can be done in front of the television, as long as you're not attempting to watch live sport or anything with a complex plot or structure.
- Drawing, or some people swear by adult colouring books. These are not colouring books with adult themes, but books containing detailed drawn designs that you have to colour in. As a creative person I find this both fiddly and dull, but they're very popular at the moment.
- Listen to something soothing and calming. New Age shops have music to meditate to, recordings of whale sounds and so on. There are also meditation apps to download for your phone, such as Calm.
- You may find avoiding social media helps. Facebook and Instagram have been proven to increase anxiety. On Instagram I tend just to follow various giant dogs, but if you're wont to look at lots of fitness bloggers or people in bikinis, maybe give social media a rest.

Mum drops me at the farm for Spin. Entering the barn, I start setting up my bike. Mum rushes into the barn.

"Quick, darling there's someone I want you to meet," she says.

Outside, there is a woman holding the most beautiful dog I've ever seen. He looks like a golden retriever but larger, with silky fur and a brown coat.

"Hello," I say. "What sort of dog is this person?"

"He's a liver flat-coated retriever," his owner says. "He's called Gandalf."

"Isn't he gorgeous," I say. "Do you need any help walking him?"

"How about Friday morning?" she says.

"I know where Iona lives," Mum says to me. "We're in book group together. I'll take you there on Friday after Spin."

"Is about ten forty-five OK?" I ask, stroking Gandalf on the top of his soft head. He gazes up at me with liquid brown eyes.

"Perfect, see you then," Iona says.

Returning to my class just as it's about to start I feel excited that I've landed a new client, and such a handsome one too.

Mum drops me at Gandalf's house on Friday. He's wearing a harness when I get there and is excited to see me: tail wagging. He brings me a slipper and drops it at my feet.

"Hello lovely," I say, giving the slipper back to Iona.

"Here's a couple of poo bags and some treats," Iona says, handing them to me. Her house is gorgeous – a large cottage with a lawn at the front and a beautiful garden.

"Where do you usually walk him?" I ask.

"In the woods," Iona says.

"Great, I'll take him there," I say, picking up the lead, putting the poo bags and the treats in my pockets.

We walk out of the gated development where Gandalf lives, and take the third right onto my parents' road. There's a gap in a fence to go through to get to the woods and we walk down the path between the trees. A blackbird hops in front of us and digs into the earth, searching for worms. A squirrel darts up a nearby tree. It's beautiful in the woods, even in winter. Gandalf walks just in front of me. He's an entire male so he scent marks everything by doing a bit of wee on it.

My friend Polly approaches with a bulldog off the lead.

"Hi Polly, he's not friendly," I say. "He's an entire male so other dogs get aggressive towards him. I'd put your dog on the lead."

She puts the bulldog on the lead; he growls and strains to approach us as we pass.

We cross a bridge over a stream – the same stream that runs along the bottom of my parents' garden – and then we're in a clearing. On our right is a fence and behind that the golf course. On our left are fields. There are some fallen trees in the clearing, so I sit on one and persuade Gandalf to sit next to me for photos. He's such a beautiful boy and so gentle.

We leave the clearing and continue through the woods until they open out into the fields. The fields are bare now it's winter. We walk along the hedgerow between the fields. Looking up, I see a buzzard circling above us: brown underside, fanned tail. We continue to where there's a hollow tree and sit for some photos there.

"Good boy," I say, handing Gandalf a treat and kissing him on the top of his head, which is so soft. I love this boy. We walk downhill to the muckheap and the walk finishes there, beyond that it's the road. So, we head back, past the fields, through the woods and back to Gandalf's house. As we enter the gate to his community, I give him another treat.

Ringing the doorbell, I wait.

"How was he?" Iona asks, opening the door. She's wearing jeans and a Breton top.

"He was such a good boy," I say. "I love him."

"He's not always a good boy," she says as Gandalf stands next to her, waving his feathery tail.

"Please may I walk him again next week?" I ask.

"Yes. Ten forty-five again?" she asks.

"Perfect," I say. "Goodbye Gandalf," I say, stroking the soft top of his head. "See you next week," I say to Iona.

"Thank you," she says to me.

Heading back to my parents' house, I feel jubilant. I've acquired a new dog client who lives nearby, and such a gorgeous one. I'm just so pleased with myself. *Things are looking up*, I think, as I return to my parentals for a bath and then lunch. Two dog clients. *Well done me*, I think as I walk down the road in the February sunshine. The air is crisp but it's sunny: perfect for dog-walking.

Chapter 30

APRIL 2017

I'm lying on a sun lounger on a large terrace, up a mountain. The side of the mountain stretches down in front of me, and mountains surround me, and there in front of me is the sea: blue and glistening. I'm in Haifa in Northern Israel with my parents, visiting my brother who's an academic at the university here. A little bird lands on the white railings in front of me. He's emerald green and metallic blue with a curved beak. He looks like a hummingbird. I sit on my sun lounger watching him and eventually he flies away.

Going inside I look up 'hummingbird, Israel' on Google and discover there's one species of hummingbird here. It's called the Palestine sunbird. So that's what I saw.

"Come on Cordelia, we have to get going," Mum says, clattering up the stairs. There's a curved wooden staircase that connects my attic room to the rest of the house. We're staying in my brother's landlord's house and it's just beautiful – all open-plan with sea views and bougainvillea around the front door and covering a canopy.

"Just coming," I say, slipping my feet into my gold sequinned FitFlops. I'm wearing my yellow Matthew Williamson at Debenhams flower print bikini covered by a matching tunic.

We pile into my brother's car. She's a Honda called Jane Honda. My brother drives us down the steep mountain roads to the beach car park and we park the car and walk along the promenade which is full of restaurants. During the British Mandate, Haifa was an important port and there was a railway line just behind the beach, parallel to the sea. So, there aren't hotels all along the beach (as in, say, Tel Aviv) and there are miles of unspoilt coastline.

We find a spot to park ourselves on the beach. Mum never goes in the sea so I leave my book and towel with her. Taking off my tunic, I persuade Mum to snap some photos of me on the beach in my bikini for the blog. Then I wade into the water, which seems cold, but I know I will get used to it. It feels so good to be swimming in the sea: I haven't done this since last April – a year ago. There are little waves and I ride them, gazing at all the colours of the sea – blue, green and turquoise – as it stretches out into the distance.

"Hello," my brother Carl says, swimming up alongside me. "This is the first time I've been in the sea this year – whenever I come down to the beach I've got my computer with me, or I've got a training session."

"Well, you're in the sea now," I say. "Let's swim to the end of that promontory."

"OK, I'll race you," Carl says.

Setting off, I'm ahead, I'm a stronger swimmer, and I win easily.

We swim a couple of loops around the bay. It is just so lovely and calming to be in the sea. Then we get out and I lie on my towel to dry off. It's hot and the sun is strong, so I put some sun cream on.

We visit one of the beach cafés for lunch. Sitting at the front, looking over the beautiful turquoise sea, I think how different I feel from this time last year, when by this time of day I would have already purchased some horrible wine from a beach bar and drunk it. Now I'm drinking Diet Coke and I feel so much better not to be an alcoholic anymore.

"Isn't this wonderful," Mum says, sipping her sparkling water. "We're all here together and …"

"Thank you for visiting me, family," my brother says, smiling at us. "It's so good to have you here."

"It's great to be here," I say.

Our food arrives – enormous salads. They certainly know how to make a salad here in Israel: it's in a huge bowl and there's grated carrots and pomegranate seeds and kale and avocado and feta and it looks wonderful.

"So, my friend runs a pottery workshop in an artists' village nearby," Carl says. "I thought perhaps I could do that, with my sister, and we could all visit the nearby Roman ruins."

"Yes, that sounds great," I say, taking a mouthful of salad and a bite of matzah. We're here at Passover, so we're not eating bread.

"You two can look around the artists' village whilst we're doing the pottery workshop," my brother says to my parents.

"OK," Mum says. "When do you want to do that?"

"How about Thursday?" Carl says. "The Roman site has only recently been excavated and there are meant to be villas with some wonderful mosaics. It's been on my list of places to visit for ages."

"Yes, let's go there," Dad says.

Dad pays the bill, and we walk back to the car along the promenade and my brother drives us back to the house. He goes off to his own apartment, just down the slope, to do some work.

Climbing the spiral staircase to my attic room I take my bikini off, rinse it in the sink of my en suite bathroom and lay it out on a sun lounger to dry in the sunshine. Closing the glass door to the balcony, I press the button to start the electric blinds descending. They're metal and when they're dropped down they plunge the room into darkness. Pressing the button to start the air conditioning, I hear the air blowing. Climbing into bed for my afternoon sleep, I close my eyes and drift off.

Chapter 31

APRIL 2017

"Wow, what a beautiful mosaic," I say. We've come to Zippori, which the Jewish historian Josephus billed as "the ornament of all Galilee". The Talmud describes it as "perched on a mountain like a bird" and "a land flowing with milk and honey for sixteen miles around".

"Yeah, I've heard people talking about it here and I've been meaning to come here for ages," Carl says. "I'm so glad you're all here with me to see it."

We're gazing at a mosaic floor which has been dubbed the "Mona Lisa of the Galilee," because it contains the image of a beautiful woman whose eyes, like those of the work of art she was named for, seem to follow you around the room. The mosaic is situated in the dining room of a wealthy late-Roman-era home that was destroyed in an earthquake in the mid-third century. Scholars don't know who lived in the house but a hint could be that the rest of the house is full of images of Dionysus and his various drunken escapades.

We troop down the ancient main street to the Nile House which possesses what I feel is an even better mosaic depicting animals, both real and imagined, from Africa. Here, it says, the inhabitants celebrated the annual flooding of the Nile.

Zippori is full of historical tales as well as its architectural marvels. According to Josephus, Herod the Great conquered the city in a snowstorm, defeating his rivals, the last of the Hasmonean rulers. In Roman times, the city was ruled by Herod Antipas and may well have been the home of one of Jesus' wealthy female disciples, Joanna, the wife of Cuza mentioned in Luke 8:3. The people of Zippori managed to escape the turbulence of the Great Revolt of the Jews against the Romans in 66 AD by opening their gates to the conqueror. After the second century Bar Kokhba Revolt, Zippori's Jewish leaders were replaced by pagans.

"Let's do a photo here," I say, when we arrive at the ancient four thousand five hundred seat amphitheatre.

"OK, then," my brother says. We climb up onto the stage and Dad takes a photo which is so good I make it my Facebook profile picture. I've lost most of the cancer weight and I'm wearing a secret support black vest top and some tiny Adidas multi-coloured shorts. I look happy, which indeed I am to be with my family at this wonderful place.

We move on to the Jewish quarter and look at the ritual baths unearthed there. This quarter was established after the Sanhedrin – the council of Rabbis – moved to the city under the famous Rabbi Judah HaNasi, who redacted the Mishnah there in around 200 AD. We look at the tomb of Judah HaNasi's grandson, Rabbi Yudan Nesiah. Then it's on to the Crusader Church of St Anne, Jesus' grandmother who, according to legend, was born at Zippori. We climb to the roof to obtain the promised bird's eye view: we can see the mountains all around us and the gigantic reservoir with its ancient aqueduct.

Last, we visit the synagogue. Built at the beginning of the fifth century AD, its prayer hall has a spectacular mosaic depicting Bible stories and Jewish symbols. Scholars have detected a note of optimism in the symbolism of the floor, built in a time where Jews were not allowed into Jerusalem by that city's Christian overlords at the time.

It's getting hot, it's nearly lunchtime, so we go to the gift shop on our way out.

"That was amazing," I say to my brother.

"Yeah, there are all these places up here in the north that people have no idea exist," he says.

"We love Haifa and the north," Mum says.

"So do I," Carl says, it's lovely to be experiencing places like this with you lot."

"Oh look, I have to have him," I say, picking up a fluffy bearded vulture. We've seen bearded vultures up in the nature reserve at the top of Mount Carmel where they breed them for reintroduction to the wild.

"I'm going to call him Vlad," I say, happy to have another stuffed toy to add to my collection. And he is a beautiful beast with his furry white neck.

Carrying my new vulture, we set off back to the car.

"There are two options for lunch," my brother says. "The posh restaurant or the traditional Arab one so …"

"Let's try the traditional Arab one," Dad says.

We set off in search of lunch, driving through the beautiful mountains, and I think how lucky I am to be in this fascinating, beautiful place with my family, my mood up, no longer an alcoholic.

"I'm having such a wonderful holiday," I say.

"I'm very glad to hear it," my brother says, smiling at me.

The north of Israel is beautiful but the Israeli tourist board doesn't focus on this region. Brother thinks this is due to the large Arab population here. Zippori, with its wonderful mosaics, and Beit Shean knock the socks off Caesarea as Roman sites, but few tourists visit them. It is a shame. Go there, dear reader, you won't regret it.

Chapter 32

Signs of Depression

- Waking up thinking, "I can't believe I'm still alive."
- Waking up late and not wanting to get up.
- Insomnia or hypersomnia or "early waking" which is waking at about three or four a.m. and being unable to return to sleep.
- Avoiding social situations. Being unable to leave the house or to make a telephone call. Crossing the road to avoid speaking to friends. Not answering the phone or calling people back or even responding to text messages or emails.
- Wearing black or dull clothes and no make-up. One of my aunts says she can always tell when my mood has dropped as I stop wearing make-up. The face takes on what is called a "flattened affect" which I think is a flat expression. When depressed I wear dark-coloured tracksuits or gym clothes – there seems no point in dressing up.
- Being unable to wash or brush hair, or in extreme cases being unable to clean teeth.
- Wearing the "dressing gown of despair" as Mary terms it.
- Feeling as if you're walking through treacle.
- Being unable to concentrate or to perform simple tasks such as cook or run a bath.
- Pushing people away yet feeling lonely.

- Feeling confused and dissociated, as if there's a pane of glass between you and everyone else.
- Cancelling arrangements you made when feeling better.
- Being very late for everything as it takes you so long to get out of the house.
- Feeling that everything will always be this way, that everything is hopeless and will remain hopeless forever.
- Loss of interest in things you've previously enjoyed e.g., food, sport, theatre, film.
- Loss of libido. Pushing your partner away.
- I feel sad and cry a lot but not everyone does. Some people don't cry at all.
- Loss of appetite or in some cases comfort eating. With me it tends to be loss of appetite, but people are different.
- Suicidal thoughts or ideation or, in the worst cases, actual plans. If you've started making plans for suicide, please tell someone. If someone has told you they're planning to kill themselves, please take it with the utmost seriousness, and don't – whatever you do – dismiss it. bipolar has a high death rate.
- You may well experience physical symptoms such as nausea, dizziness, weakness. I notice a lack of strength and speed in the gym and at Spin – I simply can't cycle so fast or with so much resistance, and I can't lift such heavy weights as when my mood is up. Depression affects the body as well as the mind.
- Confusion. Inability to carry out simple tasks or simple instructions. Forgetting plans, losing house keys and so on. In depression, connections between neurons don't get made so the brain is slowed down, and you become less capable of completing tasks.
- Being unable to stand up for oneself, due to low self-esteem.

- Losing jobs or contracts due to the inability to go to work when feeling miserable. I used to become convinced I'd be sacked from my job whenever my mood was low.

Signs of Mania/Hypomania

- Waking up early – say six a.m. – full of excitement and ready to get on with the day.
- Being charming and talkative, which soon turns to loud and obnoxious.
- Writing, smoking, talking – doing everything to excess. Being on the phone or internet or both constantly.
- Eating more or not at all. Sometimes, when my mood is very high, I forget to eat.
- Losing weight: what with forgetting to eat and rushing around full of nervous energy.
- Spending loads of money – buying silly things, up to and including cars and houses. If you're aware you're becoming hypomanic or even manic, it's a good idea to give your credit cards to someone else for safe-keeping. I know other manic depressives who have run up terrible debts when high. Dad has never let me have a credit card for this reason, so any money I spend is mine and comes out of my account, using my debit card.
- Giving houses away. I know people who have done this.
- Being creative: writing a lot, painting a lot.
- Wearing garishly coloured or revealing clothes and lots of make-up.
- Taking clothes off: either in a sexual way or because you feel really hot from too much nervous energy.
- Excessive libido, or getting into bad or unwise romantic situations with unsuitable people such as addicts, married men, teenage boys and drug dealers.

- Thinking that cars will bend round you. They won't. Possibly causing accidents in this way, or by reckless driving. If you're aware you're hypomanic or manic, please give car keys to someone else to look after until your mood has come down a bit.
- Being irritable. Feeling frustrated that other people can't keep up with your stream of thoughts.
- Seeking out social situations. It's a good idea to avoid them and to stay somewhere calm and quiet and unstimulating. My psychiatrist urges me to stay with the parentals at these times and to lie in a darkened room, away from causes of stimulation.
- Exhausting oneself. It may be a simple matter of resting in a safe environment and cutting down your dose of antidepressants will help you, or you may need to go to hospital. Hypomania and mania can cause you to be a real danger to yourself and others – this is often where the perceived glamour of mental illness comes from, someone being the life and soul of the party. In reality, mania is anything but glamorous.
- Making too many plans – which you'll cancel once your mood drops.
- Leaving jobs, telling people what you think of them and getting fired from jobs.
- Finding everything hilarious, including things that are not funny.
- Behaving inappropriately in social situations and sometimes getting yourself into trouble with friends and colleagues.
- An increase of strength at the gym, which can lead to injuries.
- Staying up late and not sleeping.
- Thinking only you know the real reality – believing conspiracy theories, suffering from religious mania.
- Aural or visual hallucinations.
- Becoming violent – maybe as a result of voices, or of frustration.

Signs of both mania and depression are not limited to the above – you may well have different ones. People experience the illness in their own individual ways, after all. I hope these have been helpful.

Chapter 33

NOVEMBER 2017

"I'm going to take some blood out of your port," the nurse says. "Then I'm going to give you the bisphosphonate injection."

"The little card that says I'm having chemotherapy," I say. "I've lost it. Please may I have another one?"

"Of course," the nurse says, smiling. "I'll be back in a minute." She's small and pretty, with freckles and hair scraped back in a ponytail, wearing the regulation bright blue uniform they wear here. I've come to the private cancer hospital for my six-monthly bisphosphonate injection. This is to seal my bones against cancer. They've been using it for a while to seal bones against osteoporosis and have recently started giving it to people with cancer in their bones, but it's very new that they're giving it to people who are just at risk of bone metastasis, like me. This treatment is not yet available on the NHS, and I only found out about it from an American chum on the Young Women with Breast Cancer Facebook group. Then I asked my oncologist for it, who supported the idea. I think recent studies have shown it has some success in preventing cancer getting to the bones.

The nurse returns with a trolley full of trays containing test tubes and plasters and dressings.

"Now, I'm just going to spray you with this numbing spray," she says, spraying it on the area of my chest where the port is. It feels very cold. "I'm just going to open the port now," she says, pushing a cannula into the port. It makes a clicking noise, and despite the numbing spray, it hurts.

"Ow," I say. "That hurt."

"At least she didn't bite you," Mum says to the nurse. "Spitfire bit me when Emma gave him his injections, and he growled at her."

"It's clever though, look," I say to Mum as I watch the blood flowing out of the port and filling one, two, three test tubes.

"Very clever," Mum says.

"What are you going to test my blood for?" I ask.

"General blood count and also tumour markers," the nurse says. "All done." She puts the test tubes on the top of the trolley and motions to open a Tegaderm dressing.

"No, she's allergic to those," Mum says.

"What about this?" the nurse asks, brandishing some white Micropore tape.

"No, she's allergic to that as well," Mum says. "She's had so much chemotherapy, it's made her allergic to all kinds of dressings. Do you have any normal plasters?"

"No," the nurse says. "We don't have any of them."

"Wait a sec," Mum says, rifling through her handbag. "I've got a couple here." She hands the nurse a plaster and the nurse puts it on me.

"I'm just going to get your implant injection," the nurse says, wheeling the trolley out.

"I can't be the only person who's allergic to all types of dressings," I say to Mum.

"I've never heard of anyone having as much treatment as you, darling," Mum says, stroking my arm. And it's true. It's been two and a half years since Mum asked my oncologist what the research said about letrozole and Zoladex's effectiveness against my particular cancer, and he told her there was no data beyond two years. So I've outlived their predictions by six months already.

The nurse returns with my injection.

"It's just a little needle," she says, jabbing it into my tummy.

"Ouch," I say. "That hurt."

"Now I just need to take your blood pressure," she says, wheeling in the huge blood pressure machine and picking up the Velcro-fastened cuff.

"I can't have it on my arm," I say. "I've had all my nodes out and ..."

"OK, we can do it on your leg," she says, fastening the cuff to my leg, putting the little clip on my finger. The numbers move on the screen, and she reads out a number.

"Is that OK?" I ask. They suffer from high blood pressure in Mum's family and I don't want that as well.

"It's perfect," Mum says.

"I just need to take a reading for your oxygen saturation," the nurse says. "Just breathe."

I take a few breaths in and out and stop talking.

"OK, that's all done," the nurse says, pulling out a sheet of paper. "Now, are you very tired?"

"Yes," I say. "Is that a side effect of the treatment?"

"Yes, it is," she says. "Constipation? Diarrhoea?"

"Constipation," I say.

"Do you take anything for it?" she asks.

"Yes, I take sodium docusate for it," I say. I've been taking this since I first started getting constipation from chemotherapy, almost four years ago now.

"Any other side effects you've noticed?" she asks.

"Well, my hair has thinned a lot," I say.

"That won't be from this treatment," she says. "That's more likely to be from the letrazole."

"Are you sure?" I ask.

She nods. "Yes, that's an effect of the letrazole. If you go to Holland and Barrett and get some multivitamins, that might help, or some vitamin A liquid to put on your hair."

"OK, we'll try that," Mum says. "Thank you."

"We need to make an appointment for you in six months," the nurse says. "So, the fourth or the eleventh of May."

"Can we do the fourth please," I ask. "The eleventh is close to my birthday and …"

"Are you worried you'll still be feeling ill by your birthday, darling?" Mum asks me.

"Well, I don't know, do I?" I reply

"OK, come on the fourth," the nurse says. "I'll just get you a new card."

She returns with a little card which says: "The bearer of this card is undergoing chemotherapy."

"Now you can just call us anytime," she says. "Here are the numbers." She points to the numbers on the card.

"Thank you," I say.

Picking up my coat and bag, putting my shoes on, I prepare to go. "See you in six months," I say.

"Don't forget, darling, call us if you have any problems," the nurse says, smiling at me.

"I will," I say.

Going down the steps and out of the building, we walk to the car.

"So, you're going to Spin after this?" Dr Stein gestures to my leggings as I sit down opposite him.

"Yes, Spin's at 9.45 a.m." I say, sitting down, putting my hands round my warm coffee cup. It's the eleventh of November and it feels cold.

"How have you been?" he asks, opening the file of my notes, pen poised above the paper.

"So, you remember my mood came up?" I ask. "It had just come up last time I saw you and I dropped my antidepressant dose down a bit."

"Yes, I remember."

"Well, I started feeling not good again: miserable for someone who wasn't meant to be depressed, so this week I put the antidepressant dose back up again."

"When was that?"

"Monday, I think, or Tuesday," I say. "And I've been feeling better since then – don't know if it's the placebo effect."

"Good. That's what I would have advised you to do had you asked me," he says, scribbling in my notes. "So, what is your venlafaxine dose now?"

"A hundred and eighty-seven point five, I think. I added the thirty-seven point five back on," I say.

"Well, I'm happy with your mood as it seems today so that seems to have been a good decision," he says. "And how are you, health-wise?"

"Well, I just had the bisphosphonate implant injection yesterday," I say. "And the nurse read out the list of side effects and it seems it's that that's causing the tiredness and, I think, the hair loss, although she says that's more likely to be the letrazole or Zoladex."

"I'm not just saying this," he says, looking at my hair. "But you seem to have plenty of hair. More than me."

"Yes, but it has thinned a lot since starting the bisphosphonates. And I find it distressing." I say.

"Well, it's unnoticeable," he says. "And how's everything going?"

"I'm walking three dogs," I say. "Going to Spin say three or four times per week. Personal training once a week and maybe another gym visit.

"I'm not really meeting people, I'm still not drinking."

"Let me just say, you've done so well with that," he says. "Are you not tempted?"

"Well, I just don't go to parties where people will be drinking," I say. "Oh, and I don't really go out at night."

"The thing about alcohol is that it's ubiquitous, I'm afraid," he says. "So, you're still on the clonazepam twice a day," he says, scribbling in my notes. "What else are you taking?"

"Venlafaxine," I say, looking out of the window where the remaining leaves on the trees are red, orange and yellow. "Lurasidone …"

"Oh yes, of course," he says. "Remind me of the dose?"

"A hundred and eleven, a seventy-four and a thirty-seven," I say.

"That's right," he says, scribbling in my notes, nodding.

"Letrazole, Zoladex, fexofenadine," I say, counting them off on my fingers. "The promethazine to help me sleep, sodium docusate, Calcichews for the bisphosphonates, bisphosphonates of course…"

He chuckles. "You must rattle," he says.

"Shall I get Mum?"

"Sure,"

Striding down the corridor to the waiting room, I find Mum. "Come on, Mum, Dr Stein wants to see you."

Back in the room, I pull up the chair next to me for Mum.

"How have things been?" Dr Stein asks Mum.

"Well, I still can't get her to do anything," Mum says, looking at Dr Stein almost pleadingly. "I thought once her mood came up she might want to do a bit more but all she wants to do is exercise and write this memoir."

"Have you thought any more about taking on any work? Or voluntary work?" Dr Stein asks me expectantly.

Shaking my head, I say: "I'm at Spin or training in the morning, I'm walking three dogs. I worked for fourteen years but now I really need this time to do the memoir."

"When are you planning to finish it?" he asks, pen poised above my notes.

"By the New Year," I say. "I want a first draft done by the end of the year and I'll start editing it in the New Year."

"I suggest we come back to this in the New Year then," he says.

"Can we make another appointment?" I ask.

"How about in a month's time," he says, looking at his calendar. "Eight thirty again?"

"Yes, that's fine. Thank you, Dr Stein," Mum says. We say our goodbyes.

Back at the car, Mum looks at me. "I've made a decision," she says. "I'm going to insist you find something to do one afternoon a week."

"I can't," I say, doing up my seatbelt. "You know I need to sleep in the afternoons."

"Well, will you try and find one more dog per week, near your flat?" Mum asks, as she pulls out of the car park, into the road.

"I have been trying," I say.

"So, try harder," Mum says, hands gripping the steering wheel tightly. "We pay Dr Stein all that money, thousands of pounds: you have to take his advice."

"I do take his advice about medication and medical matters," I say. "I don't think he understands quite how physically ill I am – how I spend about twenty hours a day in bed."

"Fine," Mum says, looking at the road ahead of her. "But I want you to promise me you'll try and find at least one more dog to walk near your flat."

"I promise," I say, as we speed through the country lanes towards the farm. *I'm looking forward to Spin today*, I think.

By September 2018 I have a new dog client – Agent Orange the Shiba Inu. She lives on Golders Green High Street just round the corner from my flat. I sit with her sometimes all day when her owners go out.

One of my Spin, Pilates and barre friends has a two-year-old golden retriever who I borrow for a dog grooming course and for the Radlett Dog Show – he's a friend rather than a client. We enter the Good Hair Day event but we're not placed, even though no one has better, silkier hair than him. It's good to borrow him for walks and cuddles – I love him so much, he's such a sweet boy.

I also have two new clients in the parental village: two ex-army explosive sniffer dogs from Afghanistan. As I throw balls for them in the garden, I wish they could tell me what they saw out there. I'm glad they're now pets, loved and cared for and not on the front line in a war zone. They're such sweet, well-trained girls, a chocolate and a yellow lab.

I pull a card or do a spread for myself every day. I love tarot so much and it is already bringing a new way of looking at the world, and new friends in the welcoming Tarot Tribe on Instagram. I'm happiest when I'm in a classroom, learning, and my tarot teacher is wonderful. Born psychic to a mother with second sight, he's been practising tarot and teaching it for more than thirty years. The course takes place at my happy haven – the Destiny Rising shop at the farm. There are eight of us on the course: mostly middle-aged women, as in everything I do. I already understand many of the meanings of the Rider Waite Tarot Deck, which is based on Egyptian, medieval Jewish and Christian mysticism.

There's the tetramorph; the four signs of the Evangelists which also represent the four elements; earth, air, fire and water. The cards are emblazoned with the sun, moon, chariots and the Wheel of Fortune. There are twenty-two major arcana cards, such as the Fool, Magician, Empress and the rest, and fifty-two are the minor arcana; swords, cups, wands and pentacles.

I purchase *The Tarot Bible* in order to study the cards, suits and their meanings at home. This book has descriptions of all cards, both upright and reversed, and describes the inherent qualities of the Aces, Kings, Queens, Knights, Pages and number cards as well as the meanings of each suit and each of the major arcana.

I studied history at Oxford from 1998 to 2001 and I am really enjoying my return to this discipline.

"Now we're going to summon spirit," my tarot teacher Niall says as we sit above the Destiny Rising shop for week two of my tarot course. Our chairs are arranged in a circle around our teacher. Paintings of fairies and mermaids in psychedelic colours line the walls. We sit on embroidered cushions with tiny mirrors sewn onto them, they give the room an Eastern vibe.

"Close your eyes, everyone, and breathe in," Niall says, his voice slow and quiet. "That's right. Let's create a space for spirit to rush into."

Breathing in, closing my eyes, I empty my mind to become a channel for spirit. Breathing out, at once I'm hot and the sweat trickles down my chest, pooling under my ribs. "Breathe in, hold your breath, breathe out," Niall says. "Now summon spirit."

Inhaling, a hot flush rushes through my body. Dolly's owner, my boss, and my dear cat Furry stand in front of me: shimmering.

"Invite spirit in," Niall says.

As I breathe in, then out, the shadow figures shift towards me. They drop to the floor, coming to rest in a seated position in front of me.

Furry's long, white whiskers stand out against the black and white of his face. It is so good to see him again: his green eyes wide. Sitting, he winds his black-and-white tail about his patterned paws. My boss crosses her legs, looking as robust as she always did in our world. Indestructible, unchanging, her face lit with a gentle smile, her hair coiffed in curls that frame it.

Dolly's owner, her strength restored, gazes at me. The frailty which beset her as she lay in her hospital bed in the living room, hooked up to oxygen, has vanished and she's the tough bird-like woman I first met in the street in Belsize Park.

Communing with my spirit guides, asking them if they're happy in the next world, they nod, shimmer, as they float above the floor. I can't see their angel wings but that doesn't mean they don't possess them. Their wings are folded behind them, I realise, as they float towards me in a gust of air.

Furry gazes at me, his tail wound about his paws. His wings, I see now, are white and he flies forward to rest under my hand. Moving to stroke the soft back of his neck, my hand meets empty space.

"Now beseech spirit to withdraw," Niall says, his voice slow and gentle. *Return, shades*, I think, and they float back on a gust of air, hovering above the floor. I'm cold now, the air rushes away from me. Spirits float back to the liminal zone. A white feather drops, spinning to the floor, circling as it falls.

"Now summon spirit to you," Niall says. *Come closer, much-loved friends*, I think, and they are borne on a gust of hot air. Sweat pools on my brow and, wiping it with the back of my hand, sitting up, I see them in front of me: a black and white, bewhiskered face and two much-loved human faces, smooth, no longer etched with lines. Ageless, my two female spirit guides stare at me with kind eyes. I bask in the warmth of their love.

"Now beseech spirit to withdraw," Niall says. *You can go now*, I think, and they float back on a stream of air, sprinkling stardust in their wake. The air is cold and rushes all over me. Pulling my cardigan around me, I shiver as the spirits are borne back to their moonlit world.

"OK everyone, you can open your eyes now," Niall says. Still shivering, I let my eyelids part. "How was that?" he asks.

"I saw them," I say. "Went hot as they approached and cold as they drew back and …"

"Me too," the woman next to me says. She too has dark, curly hair and looks to be in her early fifties. "Snap." We share a secret smile.

"So, I want you all to practise summoning spirit," Niall says, looking at us. Smiling, I return his gaze.

"When should we do it?" The woman next to me asks, shifting in her chair. "What time of day or …"

"Not in bed," Niall says, shaking his head, looking serious. "At a time and in a place where you won't be disturbed, and always on an empty stomach, so …"

"I will do it when I haul myself out of bed before breakfast," I say. "About eight o'clock and …"

"Perfect," Niall says, smiling at me. "Good. So, we just sat for a few seconds because you're all new to this but …"

"It felt like minutes," I say, crossing my arms, clutching my cardigan to my stomach.

"You will build up to minutes," Niall says, looking down at his tarot book. "Try to summon spirit a few times a day so …"

"Before meals?" I ask.

"Yes, very good," Niall says. "Let's move on to the ten of wands. What can anyone tell me about this card?"

Chapter 34

How to Lose Weight

- If you can, stop drinking alcohol. I lost around a stone, or 14lbs, pretty quickly after I stopped drinking. If you just can't stop drinking – and believe me, I've been there, then try to swap full-sugar mixers for their diet versions. Spirits and sugar-free mixers are the best things to drink for weight loss, as wine and beer contain plenty of sugar and carbohydrates. Especially beer. Ditch the beer. Also, try to have alcohol-free days every week, if you can.

- Join a gym and attend classes. You'll need to do a mixture of weightlifting and aerobic exercises. For aerobic: step, Spin and Zumba are good. So is barre. Pilates is best for mind/body connection and relaxation.

- If you can, invest in a personal trainer. I see mine once a week at the moment, but when I started, I saw her twice a week.

- Alight the bus one stop early and walk. Walk to a further away bus stop. Gradual small changes make big differences.

- Take the stairs rather than a lift. Walk up and down the escalators. If you can move – do it.

- If you're on certain antipsychotics, such as olanzapine or quetiapine, or certain mood stabilisers, such as lithium or sodium valproate (Depakote) then discuss with your psychiatrist if there is a weight neutral alternative you can try. I was on carbamazepine, an anti-epileptic used as a mood stabiliser, for years. Lurasidone, (Latuda) which is licensed for bipolar in the USA but needs to be prescribed off licence here, is the most effective mood stabiliser I've tried. Check your antidepressant is weight neutral. There are books about the drugs used to treat bipolar and their side effects. Have a look at them. Knowledge is power.

- Aim to eat plenty of fruit, vegetables and wholegrains. Fish is also good, as is chicken.

- Aim for three meals and two snacks a day. Skipping meals doesn't work and can lead to bingeing on high-calorie, high-fat foods. You don't want to be hungry. If you really can't be bothered to cook, it's fine to have a bowl of porridge with a banana or honey instead of a meal.

- Cook a big batch of soup, or stew, or whatever, on a Sunday and freeze portions in Ziploc bags to defrost when you can't be bothered to cook.

- The sandwich toaster is your friend. It can also cook eggs and vegetables. I grilled burgers in it yesterday.

- Have a look at the ingredients on the protein bars you're consuming. Some are significantly higher in fat than others. Just because they're natural doesn't mean they're low-calorie.

- Take a look at the ingredients and fat and calorie content of the foods you're eating. Low-fat foods also contain a lot of sugar, so sticking to the full-fat alternatives may make more sense. I really like fat-free cottage cheese, but it's possible you won't.

- Try to make your food look appetising by including lots of colour. Beetroot, oranges, purple sprouting broccoli. "Eat the rainbow" as the saying goes.

- Avoid fad diets or anything involving cutting out whole food groups. If you have a mental illness, for example, carbohydrates help with mood stability.

- Work with your body with regard to what time of day you exercise. I exercise best and feel most like it in the morning, and there's a school of thought that the best time to go to the gym is before you've properly woken up and realised you don't want to. But morning exercise may be impossible for you. It maybe be easier to fit a lunchtime workout into your schedule, or to exercise after work. Whatever works for you.
- If you have children, and can walk them to school, by all means do this.
- Running is great exercise and all you need is a pair of running shoes. Look online to see if there's a local running group to join. There ought to be. Or if you're a mum, take a look at This Mum Runs, set up by a mum who wanted to start running and now a huge community of running mums.
- If you're very overweight or obese it may well be worth asking your doctor about orlistat (Xenical). You take this three times a day, with meals, and it stops your body absorbing about 30 per cent of the fat you consume. I lost about six stone on it when I took it. You will need to take a multivitamin with it.
- If you're obese, gastric band surgery may be the answer. There's also a treatment where you're hypnotised to believe you've had a gastric band, which also works.
- No second helpings. I lost a lot of weight in Florence. Part of that was walking everywhere, and part of it was that, whenever we went out to eat, we could only afford one course.
- Replace full-sugar drinks with diet drinks. I get through a lot of Diet Coke. And go easy on fruit juice which is full of sugars and therefore calories.
- Join an online community such as My Fitness Pal. It has an app where you calculate how much weight you want to lose, and scan or type in everything you eat each day, and it shows you

whether you've exceeded your calorie limit or not. Generally, keeping a food diary is helpful as it shows you where you're going wrong. It was partly reluctance to write down how much I was drinking that led me, in time, to giving up alcohol.

- Don't view weight loss and healthy living as a transition with an end goal, but as a new normal, a new lifestyle.
- Realise that exercise is only tiring for a few months, then it actually gives you more energy, and that your cravings for junk food are proportional to your habitual intake of it.
- Focus more on maintaining and raising metabolism and less on caloric reduction. Find a form of exercise you enjoy and that challenges you to progress in an objectively measurable way.
- Have one cheat day per week where you eat what you want.
- It's OK to have chocolate but keep it to one small square as a treat.
- Intuitive eating. Read Mel Wells' *"Hungry for More"* and *"The Goddess Revolution"* which is all about ditching diets and listening to your body. It focuses on eating the rainbow, avoiding processed foods and protein shakes and consuming fresh fruit and vegetables. The Mel Wells Academy concentrates on falling back in love with food and focusing on self-love and acceptance of your body as it is now. Shannon Kaiser who speaks at the Mel Wells event, The Self Love Summit, says "This is not your practice life". Your life starts now, today, not once you've lost half a stone. Body positivity is about appreciating what your body can do, not what it looks like. I find this approach helpful. "The less you focus on food and weight", Mel says, "the more you can find out your life's purpose". Mel is concerned with what we are really hungry for, what our souls need. Follow your dreams now, not once you're a size eight. Take up space in the world. Change your attitude to food and weight and you'll have time to improve your life. Following the Mel Wells Self Love Advent Challenge,

a different self-acceptance theory each day from December first to Christmas has brought the goddesses into my life. We support each other in pursuing our dreams. My dream is to publish this memoir. Well done me for finding my purpose and thanks to Mel and all in the Advent Challenge, at the Self Love Summit and in the Academy of the Goddess Collective.

I hope these tips are helpful. If I can lose six stone, you too can lose weight.

Spiritual Practices Which Help Me

- Meditation: I do a 20-minute body scan before my afternoon sleep and when I'm in bed at night. You can find some on the internet.
- Daily Card Pull: Set my intentions each day by pulling a card from one of my oracle, divination and affirmation, or tarot decks.
- Affirmations: I am enough; I have all I need; I am worthy; I am strong. Repeat ten times in front of the mirror.
- Wear my chakra bracelet and carry appropriate crystals: quartz, rose quartz, selenite and fluorite.
- Walk in nature, noticing the sights and sounds about me. Walking meditation is great to centre yourself in the moment.
- Light candles.
- Have a bath.
- Drink green tea.
- Do Pilates.
- Stroke Spitfire, cuddle his soft self and talk to him whilst staring into his green eyes. Tell him all my worries. He comforts me as long as I give him enough breakfasts and lunches.

Chapter 35

What I'm about to write feels transgressive – it goes against the rules we all live by: that your girlfriends have got your back; will be there for you through thick and thin; are better than any boyfriend, and so on. I've found it to be rather different: my friends have been pretty useless since I've had cancer.

Obviously, I haven't helped myself by years of bipolar in which I've swung from, when depressed:

- Not answering calls.
- Refusing to go out.
- Refusing to respond to texts.
- Refusing to attend group events.

To, when high:

- Aiding and abetting the creation of dangerous situations.
- Telling my friends what I really think of them/their husbands/ boyfriends – usually something uncomplimentary.
- Or just telling them to piss off and leave me alone.

Anyway, I haven't helped myself with this sort of thing but, by the age of nearly thirty-four, when the breast cancer arrived, I still had plenty of friends. From where I am now at forty-one the number of people I could pick up the phone and call probably stands at … OK, we'll go through them:

- Ben – have a voicemail from him that I haven't even listened to. Bad me.
- Suzy – see her most weeks but we've missed a couple, unusually for us. She's been in Abroad. We still message every day, of course. She's a teacher and worked for about seven years at a school round the corner from my flat. She's just left that job.
- Hannah – see her every two to three weeks.
- Corey – see him about every three months. About due an arrangement with him.
- Anna – although I haven't for months, years, and we used to speak every day. She moved out of town.
- Becky.
- Phoebe.
- Liz – we were having lunch every week when she was staying in Hampstead but now she's moved to Hove.
- Julia. Married to my cousin. Adore her.
- Mary – best friend. Chat on phone most days. But she lives far away so hardly see her.

I suppose the thing with this list is that there is a group of new friends moving in to take the places of people whose friendship I've outgrown.

The larger truth of it all, I think, is that I don't fit into a category with ease, which makes it hard for my friends. I like staying in and watching TV and knitting. I'm not your typical singleton – out every night drinking, going to gallery openings and bars and having one-night stands, going to weddings and festivals and so on. In my habits, I behave more like my married chums: television box sets and early nights. Other than not going to dinner parties, my life resembles theirs far more than it resembles the lives of my remaining single friends.

Back in my teens, I really was part of a tight female friendship group with my chums Lily, Emily and Siobhan. I'm not friends with Lily or Siobhan now and see Emily once or twice a year at most. I wrote my first published novel, *In Bloom*, about our drug-fuelled nightlife adventures. But I'm not part of a close-knit female friendship group now. And it makes me sad. I feel my chums who are mums have a better social life than I do, what with play dates and NCT and so on. It's not just having children I'm missing out on, it's all the new friendships that come with them. And at the same time, I'm just not out partying with Suzy.

Writing this chapter which was meant to be about how useless my friends have been, I've actually realised that in 2020 a lot of the friendships are still there, just waiting to have life blown back into them. So, actually, I'm going to do that. I'm not depressed at the moment. I'm going to make some plans.

"Don't you want to sit on a chair, darling?" I ask Suzy.

I'm sitting on the swinging seat in my parental garden. Suzy, Hannah and Ben have just arrived. Suzy takes off her FitFlops and sits on the grass

"Oh, I'm quite happy here," Suzy says, smiling, taking a bottle of water out of her bag. "Don't want to sit on one of your cushions because of Covid."

"It's fine," I say, "we're outside."

It's Friday the fifteenth of May 2020. This is the first time I've seen my besties since early March, before lockdown.

"Thank you all so much for coming to see me."

"It's lovely to be here in your Mum's beautiful garden," Hannah says thrusting a bouquet of flowers towards me.

"It's so good to see all of you," I say, looking at my three besties. We have a Sunday chat crew where we talk to each other over WhatsApp video at 10 a.m. That's lockdown for you, you can't really see anyone apart from those with whom you are in a bubble. I'm in a bubble with my parents, Suzy lives on her own and doesn't really have a bubble. Ben and his wife, kids and mum are in a bubble, and Hannah has one with her husband and three daughters. So, it's a relief that it's a warm sunny day and we can be in the garden.

The peonies bloom: one white, one fuchsia pink. The oriental poppies are out: purple and coral and enormous. Lime green euphorbia grows out of the wall: it seeded itself there. It's stunning, we love it.

"So, what's everyone been up to this week?"

"Work," they all say at once, we start laughing. "Working" at this stage of lockdown means working from home with children, who are not at school, constantly interrupting. In Ben's case, anyway. Hannah is a key worker, so her children are at school.

"Well, who'd have thought at my fortieth at the Pembroke Castle that this would be my forty-first birthday?" I ask.

"Everything is so rubbish," Hannah says. Restaurants and shops and pubs are closed. You're not allowed out except for one walk per day. No non-essential travel. You can go on a walk with one person from another household so theoretically, Mum and Dad could walk with another couple as long as they keep two metres apart. The world appears to have gone quite mad: we're all prisoners now.

"At least I have my parents and Fluffball to be with," I say.

"I'm on my own, it's tough," Suzy says, she looks sad.

"I'm so glad you're here now, my precious." I say. "Look, blue tits on the fat balls." We have a large population of birds in the garden. At the moment I can see two blue tits, two great tits, a pair of collared doves, two magpies – two for joy – a squirrel and …

"Look, Spitfire!" Hannah says as a huge orange fluffy cat clambers out of the hedge and saunters across the orange flowerbed, then the red one, to be with us.

"Let's take a walk around the garden," I say, putting my feet back into my FitFlops. I have to lie down on the swinging chair as otherwise my back really hurts, due to the cancer in my upper spine.

Heading down the slope, we turn left at the bottom towards a bed of pink heather and blue/purple hardy geraniums. "That's Furry's rose," I say, pointing at an Iceberg rose which Mum planted over our beloved cat's ashes.

"Poor Furry," Hannah says, "he was such a great cat." He lived to the ripe old age of nineteen: a long, happy life. He used to sleep in his own bedroom. Spitfire, on the other hand, being a Ragdoll, can't be left in a room on his own. As a tiny kitten he pulled up the carpet trying to get out.

"We should make some plans to go out for walks," Ben says.

"I can't walk much," I say. "My back is so painful."

"I'm sorry, my gorgeous," Suzy says.

"It is what it is," I say. "I can still do Pilates, barre, weights and personal training, but walking is a struggle."

Mum comes out with a chocolate cake with a 4 and a 1 candle lit. They sing "Happy Birthday", which I hate. The cake is delicious: chocolate with chocolate buttercream icing.

"Great cake," Ben says to Mum. "Thank you."

"I'm so glad you're all here," Mum says. "Cordelia's lucky to have such lovely friends."

"I am," I say, beginning to get tired. The chemo exhaustion comes on at about 11.30 a.m., so I usually have lunch and a sleep soon after.

"Are you tired, angel?" Hannah asks, looking at me with concern.

"A bit," I say, "I'll sleep after lunch."

"Let's to try to book another date before we go," Suzy says.

"Weather permitting," I say, although, so far, we are having a hot, dry May.

We chat about their kids, my cancer treatment, tarot which I'm doing now. *I love my chums so much*, I think. I met Ben at sixteen, Suzy at seventeen and Hannah at eighteen: they're my oldest, closest friends. And, as I look at them in the garden, I smile. What a lovely birthday.

Mum comes to sit with us, and the greater spotted woodpecker turns up. He's so beautiful: black and white with a red head and a red patch under his tail. Today, with my besties in the garden, I feel blessed. Happiness suffuses me.

Chapter 36

Back when I was about three, I'd sit at the tiny red plastic table on a red plastic chair, telling Mum I was "doing a project". And then when I was sixteen and revising for my GCSEs, I'd copy out my notebooks in tiny writing on cards and memorise them. And I'd sit there for hours, rapt in concentration, and Mum would have to tear me away from my self-imposed revision even to eat.

And two years before that, from fourteen to fifteen, I'd be lying by the pool on holiday, writing ten pages a day, every day for a year, of my first novel. Written in pencil in spiral bound notebooks, it was a sub-Jilly-Cooper romp titled *Players* in which a sixteen-year-old girl wins the World Showjumping Championships – I drew the courses out on pages of my leather-bound Filofax – and an English tennis player wins Wimbledon, and England even win the football World Cup. The stables is also a front for a cocaine-smuggling operation and my heroine is in unrequited love with a fashion-designer-wildlife-photographer-conservationist who wears a tiger-patterned suit and is obviously gay, before I really knew what gay was. This romp runs to a thousand pencil-scribbled pages and lies, unread, and even un-typed, in a drawer. But I did it and finished it.

So, I've always written. I've always had projects. And for someone who's really an extrovert, or mainly an extrovert, it's led to a hell of a lot of time on my own, in my own head. Which hasn't been too good for me, I don't think.

Now, I have to produce a new draft of this memoir, by the end of May 2021.

I've always been attracted to boys who are loners. So the bits of the relationship when Mr X and I go to dinner parties with my chums, or when he's my plus one at events, or even when he comes to family parties, just never quite happen. And that's been a cause of sadness to me. But I never have been much good at picking men.

Have I done a menopausal side effects list yet? Here goes:

Menopausal Side Effects of Cancer Treatment

- Hot flushes: this is when all of a sudden you feel hot and sweaty, and then it's gone. It happens a lot at night and is, I think, exacerbated by a memory foam mattress, one of which I have. So, I have a fan on all the time when I'm in bed, and always have a vest top under whatever I'm wearing and can no longer wear my Hobbs cashmere knitted dresses – which is unfortunate as I have four of them and I love them.
- Weaker nails: oestrogen strengthens nails, so if you're on oestrogen-blocking medication, your nails are weaker.
- More spots: Who knows why. Maybe oestrogen makes skin clearer, although one would think that being menopausal would stop spots. But it doesn't.
- Hair loss: Have lost about two-thirds of my hair, by volume. Am on some drugs to try to help with this, but they could take six months before I see a difference. Six whole months. I thought when my hair started growing back after chemotherapy my hair problems were over, but no.
- Osteopenia and osteoporosis: This is why I'm on bisphosphonates and do weight-bearing exercise, to strengthen my bones.

- Being grumpy: see *Grumpy Old Women*. I've become much more irritable and short-tempered since being menopausal. Irritability is also a consequence of an elevated mood so poor everyone-around-me. But it's no easier being me than it is being around me.

What this section is meant to be about is the sheer mundanity, most of the time, of dealing with an illness, or two illnesses, that are chronic and life-threatening. Most of the time it's not police stations and operating theatres, electric shock treatments and chemo drips. Most of the time it's being laid low with colds and upset tummies and exhaustion and watching life drift by from bed whilst you do your best to exercise and write and keep up with Facebook and Instagram and try to eat some meals that aren't porridge and watch television and wait to feel better. Because however many positive mantras you use, a lot of life is just this: feeling ill, waiting for Better Things.

When I was going through the dramatic horrors of left-side radiotherapy – which you may remember from many thousands of words ago – my motivational song was *Better Things* by The Kinks. Better Things are much-needed now, as I feel sick due to a build-up of phlegm and know I'm going to have to do the social dance of pretending to be OK in a couple of hours. I feel a list coming on.

How to Pretend to Be OK on A Rare Evening Out

- Have an afternoon sleep to give yourself the best chance possible of being awake in the evening.
- Get an Uber or, as I'm doing tonight, a lift from a chum to make travelling easier.
- Get The Squad to meet as close to where you live as possible.
- Put some make-up on.

- And maybe a dress, although it's too cold for a dress tonight – it's zero degrees or something, in mid-August!
- Have a look at the news, at least on your phone, to have something to talk about.
- Remember to ask them how work is, how their partners and children are and so on.
- Perfect an interested look, or at least don't have an eyes-glazed-over look.
- Make sure the evening starts as early as possible for maximum leaving-early possibilities.
- Make sure you've done your work so you're not just sitting there thinking "I wish I was doing my work."
- Maybe have a wash. Am not going to as I not only had a wash but also washed hair yesterday.
- Remember to pass on brother's love.
- Don't say, "Why are two of our number having three babies this week as if they don't know we're living in the End Times?" even if you think it.
- Talk about Taylor Swift's new album, *Folklore*. And last night's tennis, which no one else will have watched.
- Talk to the smokers outside: they're always the most fascinating people.
- Ask them whether they've seen any waxwings or hawfinches yet. Chances are they won't even know what these are, but whatever.
- Talk about the situation in Hong Kong. Any mass shootings or terrorist attacks this week are other conversation starters.
- If they've all been watching *Game of Thrones* on Netflix, there's nothing you can do about that.
- Show them the eight-million-pound house you've found in Midsomer.
- Pass on love from Mary.

- Maybe wear something nice as there'll be photo opportunities for Instagram.
- Clean lenses – see above.
- Show them the cascades of manta rays in the Maldives.
- Listen to them. They've probably got all sorts of ~~dull~~ fascinating work-related or domestic problems.
- Tell them about Spitfire's weight problem and reaction to dieting.
- Fall asleep at the table and wait for Suzy to take you home.
- Make sure you've caught up on Facebook, Instagram stories, blogs-to-read so you're not thinking about these at the table.
- Maybe call Mum before you set off and before Suzy arrives so you've done that.
- Remember that in a couple of hours it will all be over, and you can go home, crank the heating back up and go back to bed.
- With your new armadillo pillow sent by brother which is so big it feels like sleeping with a large dog.
- Just focus on the fact that you'll soon be back in bed.
- Nothing lasts forever.
- Thank G-d.

Chapter 37

Ever since my bipolar diagnosis aged twenty-four, I've known having children wasn't really an option for me, so when I was younger I discussed maybe using a surrogate with Mum. And then when I got the breast cancer diagnosis I had an aggressive oestrogen-dependent tumour, so I had to start chemotherapy straight away. I couldn't freeze any eggs as that would involve pumping oestrogen into my body. And then I had chemotherapy, which probably killed my eggs. Followed by Zoladex injections to put me into the menopause when the cancer spread, plus letrozole, an aromatase inhibitor on top of that. So now I'm infertile.

I was never desperate to have children, although maybe I had a vague thought that, if the right chap came along, maybe we'd go down the surrogacy route. And when I was with Seb he didn't want children.

But now, now most of my friends have them, of course there's a part of me that feels I'm missing out. And as a writer, there's a big part of female experience – pregnancy, birth and motherhood – that I'll never experience. And, of course, it's yet another way in which I'm different from my friends.

And you'd think maybe, in 2021 where it seems the world is destroying itself, perhaps fewer people would be having children. But that's just not been the case amongst my friends, who are popping out babies in their late thirties and early forties. So there's a part of me that, yes, does feel Left Out. When I see the pregnancy photos on Facebook and see the compliments people get for their glowing pregnant bodies, I feel a twinge of envy – maybe just for the attention. And then there's the way people's lives change: new mum friends, NCT and so on. And although rationally I still don't want children, I can't stop the voice that whispers I'm missing out – as my friends record their babies' first words and first steps and write about charming things their children have said, done, written and painted. And I can't quite escape the feeling their lives are somehow richer and fuller than mine, whatever the downsides of parenting are.

There's a narcissistic component to it, of course: I'm not going to pass on my genes, my looks, IQ, love of animals and so on. I'm not going to have little people to teach to read, to take to the zoo, to drag round museums. It's another way in which my life is constricted, poorer than those of my contemporaries.

And it's not as if I've got a career to show for it: I haven't. Or even a partner to share my life with. I'm not going to have anyone to care about me if, by some remote chance, I reach old age.

The Positives of Not Having Children

- I don't have my sleep disturbed by little people. The sleep disturbance is not something I'd be able to cope with, as a manic depressive.
- I'm not going to have postnatal depression or puerperal psychosis and end up in a Mother and Baby unit, or worse. I know bipolar women who've killed themselves or damaged their babies whilst in the grip of these terrifying illnesses. So that's not going to happen.
- I'm not going to lose my size eight figure which I've worked so hard to keep.
- Or lose writing time.

- Or lose my independence by being chained to a creature totally dependent on me which controls my waking and sleeping hours.

The Negatives of not Having Children

- I'm not going to make my parents into grandparents, which I know is tough for them when their friends are talking about their grandchildren.
- I'm not going to experience a child's unconditional love for me.
- Or watch it growing up and become independent from me.

On balance, I'm happy for my friends who have children, and glad I'm not them. But it has put a strain on my friendships, as I can't be around small children because of the infection risk – small children are petri dishes for any illnesses going around and I have a low white blood cell count from all the treatment. It means I can only see my friends with children in the evenings, and I'm often exhausted by then. There's a misogynistic (I think) line of thought that if you're a woman you like children and being around them. It's difficult for my friends to understand why I don't want to hang out with them and their little bundles of joy. But I find small children So Exhausting and I can't stand the screaming, crying, mess, disorder, messy eating and the way they dominate things.

The one thing I do like about small children is reading to them. I read Patrick and Julia's son *The Tale of Squirrel Nutkin* by Beatrix Potter.

Now I've written a bit about this, I feel better about it. Such is the cathartic nature of writing. To be honest, I'm more upset that I might die without knowing the great love of a dog for me, its owner, than I am about not having children. It's just another life cycle point I'm missing, I suppose. Right: time to make some supper and get on with the blog. Glad I've got that off my chest.

WINTER 2016

I feel a bit in limbo at the moment: not working much or even volunteering. I had a couple of messages from Seb, which unsettled me, but I try to block this and him from my mind as I write.

It was a good walk with Dolly today. I love her. And yet the dissatisfaction creeps in and curls its tendrils round the edges of my thoughts, threatening to break apart the fragile balance of my mood. It's just 4.34 p.m., but already dark and I do hate this part of winter. I hate the later part too, but this year we weren't gifted an Indian Summer in September and October as sometimes happens: as happened, in fact, the year I bought my flat when I remember parading about in hotpants until well into October.

Anyway: I know now that someone is waiting to read my book – two people in fact. I've known them for sixteen years or thereabouts – I had my first job at their agency. I was a different person then, and it was another world – the early noughties: long, boozy client lunches; publishers' parties all the time; trips to Bologna Children's Book Fair in April. It was a carefree time that ended in a four-day bender and six weeks in the mental hospital with psychosis. Anyway, I'm glad they're looking forward to the book. I'd better make it good.

I am trying to make it good. I've been doing a little thought experiment: if I was someone else and just catapulted into my life, what changes would I make. Here are some I've come up with:

Changes I Would Make

* Let the spare room at the flat. It would bring in some much-needed cash and also provide me with some human company. I don't feel well enough to do that at the moment, partly because I spend so much time in bed and watching television in the

living room in my sleepwear, but that's probably where I'd start. So, the goal is to become well enough to get out and about a bit more, with the eventual result of arriving at a place where I feel well enough to have someone else renting the spare room. This would also involve fixing the broken things in the flat.

- I could fix the broken things in the flat, sell it, and buy a small house close to my parents where, maybe, I could have a dog. If I could find a small house close to my parents, that is. Small houses are in short supply round there as bungalow owners tend to be selling their houses which are then knocked down and massive houses with tiny gardens are built on the plots.
- Take up driving again. If I could pass a driving test, then I could look for a small house near my parentals and would be able to drive to Spin and to the shops and to take my future dog to the vet.
- Retrain as something: maybe a personal trainer.
- Visit my brother in Abroad.
- Publish a book.
- Wear wigs.
- Really throw self into the dating.
- Make a separate Instagram account for Spitfire to maximise opportunities there.
- Go out more.

At the parentals I have company and I'm busier, with Spin, barre, Pilates and walking Gandalf. I sleep better at the parentals, but I don't really see people apart from them and Spitfire, unless Mum invites people over. When they go out, I stay at home with my cat. I suppose I feel I'm living two half-lives, rather than one integrated one. When I first lived at this flat about seven years ago, I used to spend more time here. But then I also had flatmates, no cancer diagnosis, a job three days a week and my friends hadn't started procreating, so I saw more people. I used to go out drinking, to bars and pubs, out to parties, into town.

Most of my problems are related to having a chronic life-threatening illness, a chronic mental disorder and no partner. It's a stage of life thing. When my uncle was single and in his thirties and early forties he was involved with his synagogue, and I did try that when I was about thirty-one, but this flat is too far away from that synagogue, and to be honest that one has an ageing population.

2021

Now I'm busy rewriting this memoir, being a published author and professional tarot reader and studying astrology. My life is unrecognisable from what it was in 2016: I've found happiness in what I do for money and my studies.

"Do you want me to pull you a card?" I ask Mary whilst we're on our daily, sometimes two or three or four times a day chat.

"Oh yes, and I'll do one for you," she says.

We started our tarot and oracle Instagram accounts about eighteen months ago. I trained – did a beginners' tarot course at my local holistic shop, Destiny Rising, followed by an advanced tarot diploma at the Centre of Excellence. She started designing her own animal oracle deck, which is beautiful and magical, but not quite finished.

I pull a card. It's the ten of cups.

"Ten of cups," I say. "It's the family card from the Tarot Illuminati, my new deck from Leon. There you are with long silver hair, with your husband in a jerkin and tights, with your two beautiful children: twins, a boy and a girl, and look at your gorgeous little house and …"

"Photograph it and send it to me." Mary says.

She receives the photo and laughs, "I love my house," It's a cottage with ivy climbing up the walls, idyllic.

"Look at your dress," I say. It's a long evening dress. "So, you're going to find a man and be happy."

"Now let's do yours," she says. "Trees or fairy-tale?"

"Fairy-tale please," I say, looking over the garden where I can see the pair of collared doves, two magpies, a great tit on the feeder. The bullfinch flies in, a burst of blue and red and perches on the water bath.

"Bullfinch." I say.

"You're so lucky," Mary says. "I'd love to get a photo of him."

"He's already gone," I say. "He doesn't feed at the feeding station, just flies in for a bath."

"So, yours is the eight of swords from the fairy-tale deck. Oh no, I'm sorry," she says. "I'll send it to you."

It arrives. It's a girl, crying in bed, with eight swords at the end of the bed. She is hugging a fawn.

"I wish I had my own fawn," I say, feeling sad. Chemo starts again in a few days and I'm not looking forward to being ill and perhaps bedridden from it.

"I'm sorry, darling," she says.

"Cordelia," Mum's voice rings out. "We're going in ten minutes, are you ready?"

"Almost," I shout back. "Right, darling, I'd better go, talk to you later."

"I'll never forget you," Mary says.

"I'll call you later, bye, love you." I say.

"Love you," Mary says, and the line goes dead.

When I did my tarot course at Destiny Rising, we learnt on the Rider Waite deck, the original English deck published in December 1909 by Rider Waite and illustrated by Pamela Colman Smith. This deck quickly caught on and is now the standard English deck: many new decks, and there are thousands, are based on its imagery.

My teacher took us through the history of tarot – invented in the 1400s in Italy – the Visconti-Sforza deck and the Minchiate Etruria from Florence, up to the present day. We learnt each of the major arcana cards such as The Moon, Strength, The High Priestess and their meanings. Then on to the suits of wands, cups, swords and pentacles. Each suit represents an element: wands are fire, cups are water, swords are air and pentacles are earth. Each of the major arcana, meanwhile, corresponds to a planet or star sign: The Moon is Pisces, Justice is Libra, The Lovers are Gemini, whilst The Wheel of Fortune is Jupiter, The High Priestess is The Moon and The Magician is Mercury.

There are seventy-eight cards, twenty-two major arcana and fifty-six suit cards. You shuffle them and draw a spread to answer a client's question. There are career, love and destiny spreads.

I had set up my Instagram as @Unique_Unicorn_Tarot, but changed the name to @TaurusSunAndMercuryTarot as the more astrology I learnt, the more I incorporated into my readings. I recommend Corinne Kenner's *Tarot and Astrology*, Brigit Esselmont's *Intuitive Tarot* and Mary Greer's *How to Interpret the Tarot Court Cards*. These three books have really helped me. Every day I use my copy of *The Tarot Bible* by Sarah Bartlett.

I have acquired many tarot clients by word of mouth and have worked through March, April and May this year.

Last October, I started a three-year astrology diploma at the London School of Astrology. It's wonderful. After two terms I've already learnt so much. I can cast a chart, know about decans and signs, the glyphs for the planets, transits, chart shapes. I've also attended two astrology weekend courses run by the London School of Astrology and the Mayo School.

Before the degree, I did two Centre of Excellence diplomas in astrology and medical astrology, which I loved. If you want to learn astrology I recommend picking up *The Astrology Bible* by Judy Hall in the Godsfield Bible series. If it sparks your interest, do a Centre of Excellence course and then look at the London School of Astrology website: it's really informative, I'm enjoying it so much.

Tarot and astrology have changed my life. They give some structure and meaning to all the randomness. I love reading about them and practising them and I can't recommend them enough as ways of finding out about yourself, your behaviour, your motivations, as well as relationships and how others tick: their blind spots, the aspects of them which frustrate you and so on.

Chapter 38

Music That Helps Me

- Leonard Cohen
- The Kinks
- Taylor Swift
- ABBA
- George Michael
- Blondie
- Nick Drake
- Portishead
- The Doors
- Absolute Radio 90s – for all my nineties favourites
- Britney Spears
- Robbie Williams
- Orbital
- The Orb
- New Order
- Happy Mondays
- Emily DiPace
- Lemon Jelly
- Queen
- Taylor Swift

Chapter 39

"Do you want to hold them?" Gemma asks. We're sitting on her big sofa, downstairs in her flat. Gemma is expressing milk using a breast pump and her partner Mike has just walked downstairs with the new twins.

"Yes, please," I say, opening my arms.

Gently, Mike puts a little boy in my left arm and one in my right. The one on the right is awake and his eyes are as blue as a kitten's. They were born just a week ago.

"Hello, little chap," I say, looking into his eyes. He grasps my thumb with a surprisingly strong grip.

"Can he see me?" I ask.

"I think he can see about twenty centimetres away, in black and white," Gemma says. The breast pump whirrs.

"They're amazing," I say. The little boys just lie there, warm and tiny. It feels profound, this moment. I've never liked babies but maybe I just haven't met the right ones before, because these two are wonderful.

"So, how are you finding it?" I ask Gemma.

"This thing is annoying," she says, gesturing to the breast pump. "It takes about forty-five minutes to get a bottleful, but the boys are amazing."

"They're beautiful," I say, looking at their tiny perfect heads, covered in downy dirty blond hair, their little hands. They warm me up – two mini hot water bottles.

"I wanted to see how you are," I say. "I thought you might be really freaking out or …"

"I've had a couple of meltdowns," she says. "But it's been surprisingly OK and …"

"Have you been out and about anywhere yet?" I ask, looking into the pair of tiny blue eyes. He looks at me, I'm sure he does.

"Not yet – my caesarean scar hasn't healed yet," Gemma says. "It still hurts."

"I'm not doing much at the moment," I say. "I can come every week – Monday or Tuesday or …"

"Why don't you come on Mondays," Gemma says. "My Mum's coming on Tuesdays." At last some milk is flowing, slowly, into the bottle. The pump makes a relaxing humming noise.

"I'd like that," I say, smiling at her. *A new start*, I think, *with two new babies. What a lovely thing to happen*. And I feel really happy. Well done me.

Chapter 40

MAY 2018

I'm walking to my polling station from the flat and I can't breathe. I just can't catch my breath. Sitting down on the wall outside the church, about five hundred metres from my flat, I try to suck some air into my lungs but can't. I'm frightened. I know this isn't a panic attack.

Crawl, almost, up the tiny incline across the road. Stop again. Can't pull any oxygen out of the air. Stand up, dizzy. Resting my hand against the fence, I turn into the school grounds – the local school is the polling station today. Creeping up the slope, I sit down again on the circular wooden bench around the oak tree at the edge of the school playground.

Outside, the counters sit.

"Who will you be voting for?" the Conservative one asks me. Staring at his blue ribbon, the words won't come out.

"Yes," I say at last. "I can't breathe." He's a handsome chap in his thirties.

I'm now thirty-eight.

"Can I help?" he asks as I breathe frantically.

"Please," puff, puff, puff. "I'm sorry." I choke on the lack of oxygen. "Help me inside." I splutter and cough.

"There, there," he says, looking awkward. I hold his arm as he almost drags me in.

I give the teller my address sitting on the floor.

"Are you, I mean, can you …"

"Yes, I have to." Rest on ground. Breathe in but no air goes in.

She hands me a ballot paper and I put a cross in a box. Hauling myself up from the floor, staggering to the box, I push in my folded bit of paper.

Then it's the ten-minute walk back to the flat. Somehow, I make it, stopping on the wall outside the school, the wall in front of the church. Somehow, I'm sitting on the front step of my block of flats, gasping for air, a fish out of water.

Crawling across the bridge, I collapse into the lift. I press the button, sitting on the lift floor. We descend to lower ground. Sitting outside the lift, I scramble in my bag for the keys. Find them: success. Open flat door, collapse in hall of flat, can't breathe, can't breathe, can't breathe.

Text Dad. "Please come and get me, I can't breathe." Lying down on my bed, I close my eyes.

"We'd better do a scan." My oncologist says as I sit with Dad in his office. He looks worried.

"What is it?" I ask.

"I fear the cancer may have reached your lungs. Try to rest and I'll fix you a scan for tomorrow."

"Thank you," Dad says.

The walls are white, they hurt my eyes.

Dad picks up my bag. "Let's go home," he says.

At home, I lie on my bed on my back so as not to constrict my breathing further.

"Do you want to watch a Poirot?" Mum asks. "It will take your mind off tomorrow's scan."

I nod.

Mum lifts my pillows up and, holding her arm, I let her lead me through two doors to the sofa, where I collapse again.

"It will be OK, Angel," Mum says. "I love you, and so do Dad and Fluffball."

I fiddle with the remote control. Oh, here it is, the Peter Ustinov *Death on the Nile*. Soon I'm lost in it. As Poirot boards the boat to cruise down the famous river, I'm transported into another world.

"So," my oncologist says at our next meeting. He looks worried. "The cancer has spread to your lungs."

I start crying, small tears at first and then rivers down my face.

"What does that mean?" I ask, gazing over his head and out of the window behind him. It's spring and the trees are festooned with lime green for this new season.

"Well," he says, "Come and have a look."

He turns his computer on. "Here, you can see your lungs, and you notice the grey material."

"What does ... I mean, what is it?"

"The fluid fills your lungs, that's why you can't breathe. I'm afraid the cancer, which is diffuse over the surface of each lung, is producing the fluid."

Switching off, I gaze at the grey filling my lungs.

"The cancer is in the pleural membranes," he says. "We need to drain your lungs, and then you will need an operation."

Despite the unbearable pain I feel if I try to swallow, or walk uphill at all, I just can't manage, but worst-case scenario is ... no, best not to think about this.

"I'm just going to get some fluid out of your lungs. This is going to come back, but before the operation your lungs need to be empty, so it is best if we drain them now."

"Will it hurt?" I ask, looking at him. He is a handsome chap, my lung doctor: sandy brown hair and green eyes.

"Sit still and take your top off please," he says, pulling the curtains around the bed. Behind the curtain I look down at my cancer-filled chest cavity. I take off my vest top – it's a hot spring day.

"OK," I say. "How exactly will this happen?"

"Sit up for me," he says. I'm collapsed on the bed. Imagining there's a string dangling down, I pull it and I'm sitting up.

"Now take a few deep breaths; yes that's right. Needle coming now."

A sharp pain which goes on and on.

"Good girl," he says. "Be brave."

I want him to spot how exhausted I am.

"Nearly done," he says. Then a sharp stabbing pain when the needle comes out.

"All done." he says.

"So, who will do the operation?" I ask.

"There's a doctor, Charlotte, at Harefield which is a chest hospital. I'll make an appointment with her and she'll call you."

Chapter 41

"So," Dr Charlotte says. "We're going to put a drain in."

"I hate drains," I say, remembering Fluffball chasing the tube of the drain bottle when he was a kitten.

"Mum won't allow me to be sent home with a drain." I say.

"We won't let that happen," she says.

"We will repeat the process for the other lung at a later date."

"Thank you," I say, sitting up in my hospital bed.

"I'll come and check on you later." Dr Charlotte says. "They'll be here to take you down to theatre in a few minutes. You're not strong enough to walk, so we'll wheel your bed into the theatre."

"Name, date of birth." The porter says. I rattle them off.

Through many doors my bed is wheeled to the theatre dressing room. But I'm not pulling on a velvet dress to play Anne Neville.

"I'm going to count to five," the anaesthetist says. "One, two, three …"

I pass into a deep sleep.

"Where are my glasses?" I ask, on waking. I'm in excruciating pain. "I need some morphine."

"Here you are," the nurse says, squirting a syringe of Oramorph into my mouth. It tastes amazing. I open my eyes, a nurse hands me my glasses and now, miraculously, I can see.

All around me are people breathing oxygen from cylinders. Others are still sleeping.

"I want my mum, can you call her?" My speech is slurred.

"OK," she says, and strides across the room, disappearing as the bright white wall swallows her.

Maybe this is heaven, or hell. The Oramorph makes me feel less anxious. I float, a green spirit over the hills.

I don't float. I lie in bed until the porter arrives to wheel me back to the world.

Back in my room I press the bell and a nurse comes in.

"Lunch," I say. It's a struggle to get any words out as I'm drowsy from the drugs: morphine, codeine and too many others to remember.

There's a knock on the door.

"Lunch," the kitchen person says and hands me a cheddar and onion sandwich.

The pain is unbearable on the left side of my body. I step out of bed to go to the loo, but I'm dizzy and collapse on the floor, tangling the tube of my drain bottle. I struggle to my feet, there's a knock on the door.

"The door's open." I whisper, trying but unable to speak louder.

"Hello, darling." The nurse says, wheeling a huge trolley. "Let me sort you out." She untangles the tube of my drain and helps me into bed. She takes my blood pressure, which is OK, but my oxygen saturation is still very low.

"My drain site hurts," I say.

"I don't understand," I say

"Hello," a new doctor visits me. "Your surgeon isn't here today, so you've got me. I'm afraid we couldn't do the pleurodesis as your lung is completely collapsed. We are going to send you home with a drain."

"But Mum won't have me home with a drain bottle," I say.

"Nevertheless, you will go home with the drain. Our hope and expectation is that over the next two weeks your lung will inflate, now we have drained the fluid."

"Mum won't be happy," I say. "Nobody told me this might happen."

"Your lung specialist drained three and a half litres of fluid from this lung," he says, looking down at his clipboard, making notes. "We won't send you home with the drain bottle, just the tube."

"How will that work?" I ask.

"Well, too much of the lung was completely collapsed. If it reinflates, in two weeks we will attempt the operation," he says. "Meanwhile, the district nurses will come every couple of days to collect the fluid."

At home, the district nurses come every other day to change my leaking dressing and to collect the fluid which has accumulated. So much fluid spills out of my lung that the dressing is soaked every morning, and I wake up in a puddle of water.

"This is so humiliating," I say to Mum. "Am I going to have this awful thing in my side for two weeks?"

"I think the drain site is infected," Mum says, "It feels hot."

"But my surgeon said it wasn't infected." I say, looking up at my violet ceiling.

"It is infected: look." Mum pulls up my top, I can see the drain site is red and there is pus coming out.

"Yes," I say, "It hurts."

A face appears around the door. An orange face with a stripey head.

"Come in Fluffball," Mum says. He steps over all the mess, jumps up on my bed and lies there, purring.

"I love you, my precious angel," I say, stroking under his chin. He sighs and stretches his head forwards, closing his eyes.

"The district nurse will be here soon." Mum says.

I fall asleep on my front, Fluffball on the end of my bed.

"Sweetie, someone has come to see you." Mum says, sitting on the end of my bed, stroking my face. "It's Rose, who's come to drain the fluid."

Rose strides in brandishing a plastic cloth.

"This is called a rocket drain," she says, clipping it to the end of the tube.

Feeling a sharp pain as the rocket launches, dislodging the fluid, suddenly I'm crying.

"It's just so bloody unfair," I say to Rose and Mum. "Am I going to have this for the rest of my life?"

My sheet is soaked with fluid.

"All done," Rose says, unscrewing the bottle, taping the plastic tube round itself, putting a new, dry dressing over it, taping it with pink Micropore.

Walking down Beech Avenue, I despair. The panther is here, strolling along beside us.

"What is it, sweetie?" Mum asks, "Why aren't you saying anything?"

She looks at me, her eyes full of pity. I hate it when she looks at me like this. We pass the house where the house martins live as they swoop in the sky and back up to their nests in the eaves.

"Look up, sweetie." Mum says. I look up.

"The house martins are back," Mum says, putting her arm around me.

"I can see them," I say. "What if I'm like this for ever?" I ask as I feel the panther's soft head beneath my fingers. "What if I have a drain tube in for the rest of my life?"

"You won't," Mum says, "Your lung will reinflate once the fluid has gone." She pulls me closer to her.

"Good news," my lung surgeon says, as I sit with Dad in her office two weeks later. " Your lung has reinflated so we can try the operation again. Come in on Monday."

"That's great news," I say, smiling. The panther slumbers at my feet, his chin resting on one paw. He opens an amber eye and gazes up at me.

"You will never recover."

I will, I think, as I sit next to Dad in the Mercedes on the ride home. The panther is sprawled along the back seat, gazing up at me as I turn around to look at him. He stares into my eyes with his amber ones, and then closes his eyes, his head sinking down onto his paws.

"So, we are going to operate today," the surgeon says. "We will give you a general anaesthetic and, when you come round, your lung will be stuck to your chest wall with a thin layer of talcum powder between them."

"Will that stop it collapsing again?" I ask, sitting up in the hospital bed, feeling weak and exhausted.

"Yes," she says. "The talc will irritate the lung and it will remain inflated."

"That sounds like a miracle." I say.

The wren of anxiety flutters up from my stomach into my windpipe and then she is flying around the room. I watch her as she circles the ceiling above my bed. The panther lies on my legs. He doesn't notice the wren; she is too small to be even a snack for him.

"We're putting you under now," the anaesthetist says.

I'm in the tiny anteroom of the operating theatre. There's a cannula in my foot.

"Just think of your happy place," he says. "Here, give me those." He gestures for me to remove my glasses. I've already taken out all my piercings and am wearing a horrible pink-checked, open front hospital gown.

I think of being with my brother in Abroad, the waves crashing against the shore. And then, nothing.

"The operation was a success," a doctor says, as I wake up. He is tall with black hair and brown eyes.

"I need a wee," I say. *He's very handsome*, I think.

"Let me just get a couple of nurses," he says.

"We were able to complete the pleurodesis, your left lung is now inflated and good as new."

"Thank you so much," I say, feeling relieved.

"There's still a drain in, as you can see," he says. I feel down my side and there is a drain tube coming out.

"We'll keep that in while the wound drains and it will come out before you go home in about eight days' time."

There's a knock on the door and two nurses come in.

"Come on, sweetie," they say as the doctor leaves.

"Bye," I say.

"See you tomorrow," he says. "I'm George." He pulls the door shut behind him.

"Let's get you out of bed, no, not like that, you'll hurt yourself." The nurse says. She unties my drain bottle from where it's clamped to the side of the bed.

Staggering to my feet, groggy from the anaesthetic, I stand up, leaning against the bed. I breathe, deeply.

"Let's go into the bathroom," pretty nurse two says. I read her badge; she is called Poppy.

"Thank you, Poppy,"

Leaning on Poppy and the other nurse, Felicia, we make slow progress towards the bathroom. I sit on the loo, Poppy wheels my morphine drip beside me which is connected to a cannula in my foot. On the loo, nothing happens.

"Sometimes, the general anaesthetic and morphine stop you being able to evacuate your bladder," Poppy says.

I sit. And sit. Eventually a trickle of wee comes out.

"Good girl," Felicia says. She is short with blue eyes and brown hair. "Let it all out."

"I need a wash," I say, flushing the loo.

"We'll just put you back to bed first." Poppy says, flashing her white teeth as she smiles.

"It's lunchtime now, so why don't you have your lunch? We've ordered you an egg sandwich."

"Yum," I say, feeling hungry all of a sudden. Poppy reties my drain bottle to the bedframe. I press the button on my morphine drip.

"You're not to overuse that, as we'll take it away," says Felicia, sounding stern. "See you after lunch."

"Bye," I say as they leave.

Chapter 42

A herd of mammoths trundle across the screen.

"Earth was once roamed by giants," Dr Alice Roberts says. "Welcome to *Ice Age Giants*."

"I love this programme, I love Dr Alice," I say to my brother, Carl. He's visiting me in hospital. His term has ended so he caught the first flight from Abroad to see me.

"She's got rather a breathy delivery," Carl says. "Do you need something? A cup of coffee?"

"Yes please," I say, pressing the pantry call button.

"One pot of coffee to room 16 please." I say.

"Be with you in a minute," the voice says at the other end of the line. The pantry is where the magic happens, the staff are so lovely.

"One pot of coffee coming up."

"Do you want anything?" I ask my brother.

"No Cord, it's fine," Carl says. "I'll go down and get a cappuccino from the restaurant later."

"The woolly rhino also roamed the ancient earth." Dr Alice says, as we see a herd of huge rhinos, covered in long, thick, brown fur.

There's a knock on the door.

"Come in," I say.

"Just come to do your checks," the nurse says. She's a really pretty young girl – mid-twenties, I'd say. She's my favourite nurse. I recognise her voice.

264

My brother springs up out of his seat to get the door.

"Hello," Poppy says, looking at my brother. He's a striking specimen – big grey eyes and a mop of shaggy, dirty blond hair.

"Hi, I'm Carl," he says, smiling at her. "I'm Cordelia's brother."

"She's been talking about your visit," Poppy says, wheeling in the machine.

"Let me help you," Carl says, always the gentleman.

"I can manage, but thank you," she says, smiling at him.

My brother has this effect on people. He's endlessly kind and empathetic.

"Right, let's see how your oxygen saturation is," Poppy says to me. "Just put your finger in here." She clicks open a familiar plastic device. "Ah, good girl," she says looking at my bare nails. "No nail polish, this will give us a more accurate reading."

Beep, beep, beep goes the machine and then a number flashes up: 89. It's meant to be as close to a hundred as possible.

"Put your oxygen on," Poppy says, handing me a plastic tube connected to the wall behind my bed. I plug one end into my nose with the band of plastic tubing around my head. My breathing feels much easier.

So, where have you come from, Carl?" Poppy asks. "Leg please, Cordelia."

I stretch a leg out from under the covers. *I'm so tired*, I think, *it must be all the morphine, or the general anaesthetic has not worn off or …*

Waking up with a start, I see my brother next to me, reading a book. Taking the oxygen tube out of my nose, I push the lever until the back of my bed is upright.

"You had a nice long sleep," my brother says, smiling at me. I love my brother so much.

"Tired," I say. "Must be the after-effects of the operation."

"Yes," Carl says. I see he's sipping coffee from a plastic cup. A lock of his blond hair tumbles over one eye and he pushes it back.

"It's tiring, having operations. What do you want to do now? I have to get back to the parentals to get on with some work."

Carl teaches English literature at a university in Abroad. He's always writing conference papers, marking exams, reading plays, writing articles. He's such a busy person.

"Thank you for visiting me," I say. My speech sounds a bit slurred. It could be the morphine, or it could be something else. I'm not sure.

"Does my voice sound weird?" I ask. Now I'm awake, my drain site is extremely painful.

"Your speech is a bit slurred," Carl says, looking concerned.

"I'll ask a nurse when someone comes in for checks." I say.

"Dad will be along later with a film," Carl says, putting his book in his leather man-bag. "I'll see you tomorrow." I reach out my arms to hug him and … ouch … pull against the drain.

"Did we miss the rest of *Ice Age Giants*?" I ask.

"I'm afraid so, but there's a Marple on in ten minutes."

"Oh good, Marple is my best one apart from Poirot." I love Agatha Christie: the formula, the characters, the attention to the 1930s aesthetic. "Which one is it?"

"*A Caribbean Mystery*," Carl says. "See you tomorrow, sister." He puts his arms around me and then walks out.

"Wait," I shout after him, "You left your laptop." I can see it on the floor next to the chair on which he was sitting. He shakes his head and laughs.

"You'd lose your own head if it wasn't stuck onto your body." I say.

"I'm not a no-neck monster," Carl says, picking up his laptop and striding out of the door.

I feel sad and bereft now he's gone, so I switch on ITV3 and, suddenly, I'm in the Caribbean with Miss Marple and a gang of murderers on the white sand against the turquoise sea.

PART THREE

Chapter 43

MARCH 2020

"I don't want to know if there's cancer in my spine." I say to the oncologist. "Just don't tell me."

We're sitting in his office. Bare branches behind us.

"I'm afraid there's cancer in your spine," he says.

I burst into tears; the nurse puts her arms around me. I have been suspecting this. I've had a constant pain in my upper back that hasn't gone away – obviously nothing muscular.

"We're going to start you on some more palliative chemo," he says. "It will be two weeks on, one week off."

"OK," I say. "Will I still be able to exercise?"

"Of course," he says.

"Thank you." I say, disentangling myself from the nurse. I know the trajectory of breast cancer is lungs, spine, brain. I knew, deep down I knew.

The first chemo drug I try is not a success. I get a temperature the next day and get taken to A & E. This happens twice. In hospital I am given antibiotics and paracetamol and I stay in for about three days. After the second time, Mum decides she can manage to look after me at home with paracetamol, and this happens after the next two treatments. My next scan shows that the cancer has spread in my bones, lungs and liver.

"So, what's next?" I ask my oncologist.

"There's a drug called GemCarb which a few patients of mine are on – gemcitabine and carboplatin," he says. "Let's try it. One week of both drugs, one week of gemcitabine alone, then one week off." He scribbles in my notes.

I start the GemCarb and all goes well for a few months. I'm able to exercise, publish my novel, do my astrology course. I'm so relieved we have found something I can tolerate.

"So," I say to my agent in the September after the first lockdown. "I've decided I would like to publish *In Bloom*.

"That's a great idea," she says.

"I just want to get it out there," I say "before I'm too ill to enjoy it."

"Absolutely," she says. I'm on the telephone, looking out of my bedroom window. I can see robins bobbing on the ground and a great spotted woodpecker on the peanuts.

"How much will it cost me?" I ask her.

"Let's see," she says. "I'll speak to my colleague and let you know, but roughly …" She names a figure.

"That's fine," I say. I've saved up a little money due to lockdown and being on chemo. I'm shielding so I'm not allowed to leave the house.

"Let's do this," my agent says. "Let's show those publishers what they're missing."

The next day, my other agent calls with a figure. I transfer the first chunk of money and am so relieved that finally, this book will see the light of day.

I wrote *In Bloom* between the ages of twenty-five and twenty-eight, working on it during my Creative Writing MA at Birkbeck. My agent sent it out fourteen years ago but no publisher wanted it, so it was put on a shelf. But now, as I feel the end of my life approaching, I breathe life into it. I rewrote it in 2018 so by September 2020 it is definitely ready to go.

I ask my best friend Mary to make some colour illustrations and then sit back and wait. My brother's friend has just published a novel in a typeset font I like so I ask him what it is called and tell my agents so they can tell the designer.

The whole process seems astonishingly fast. By October I'm with Mary in Suffolk for the weekend and we walk round a lake with her new dog.

"There," Mary says, as I sit on a bench, unable to shield my eyes from the sun. "Just a few more." I gaze at the camera, eyes narrowed. Click, click, click goes the camera button.

"These are wonderful," Mary says, looking at them on the camera screen. "Look."

I look strong and single-minded, orange wig catching the light. "I love them," I say. "But my eyes are so narrow."

"Makes you look determined," Mary says, putting the camera back in its bag.

We turn a corner and there are my parents on a bench, gazing at the lake.

"Ah, so this is the new dog," Mum says. "Isn't she sweet? She's smaller than our Fluffball."

"She is quite small," Mary agrees.

I stroke the dog's soft head.

"She seems to like you," Mary says to me.

"I like her," I say looking at her foxy face and her big brown eyes.

"Hello, little sweetheart," Mum says, stroking her.

We walk around the lake, through the woods and up to the cemetery and arrive back at the main road of Debenham.

"I'll see you soon," I say to Mary, not knowing when I'll see her, due to this beastly Coronavirus pandemic.

"At least we were able to meet yesterday and today," Mary says. We gaze at each other.

"Come on," Dad says, opening the car door for me.

"Bye," I wave to Mary, and she waves back. My last sight of her is standing by the road, with her little dog, waving.

In Suffolk, that evening, I choose the cover from two possible options. It's black with *In Bloom* embossed on it using one of Mary's light paintings. I'm so happy with it. This is the brilliant thing about high-end self-publishing: you can choose your illustrator and cover design.

Back home, we start working on the press release. My lovely aunty, who is a journalist, agrees to help my agent with this. When it comes out it's just wonderful.

Please purchase a copy of *In Bloom*. It's literary young adult issue fiction, set in the mid-90s trance clubbing scene and is semi-autobiographical. So far, we have forty-three five-star reviews on Amazon and more are coming up all the time.

The book is ready to go by November.

"Why don't you record an audiobook?" my agent says.

This has always been a dream of mine. I find a studio in Watford and book the first three hours.

"That was word perfect," my sound engineer says. He's about my age but wearing a pinstripe suit which makes him look younger.

"Thank you," I say. "I really enjoy reading out loud."

"You're really good at it", he says, as we stand in the studio's reception area, where the walls are lined with guitars.

"And it's really funny," he says. "You had me in stiches in there. I had to turn off the feedback microphone as I was laughing so much."

"Ah good," I say, "I do want it to be funny."

"It certainly is," he says, a smile in his brown eyes.

"So, twelve till three next week?" he asks.

"Yes, perfect," I say, feeling so proud of myself for achieving my dream.

Chapter 44

"I'm afraid I've got something to tell you," Dad says as he picks me up from the flat on the eighteenth of October. "Fluffball didn't come home last night."

"What?" I ask, uncomprehending, looking at Dad's serious countenance.

"Mum called him in the late afternoon as usual and we were looking for him all evening and there was just no sign of him." Dad says, picking up my pink rucksack. My whole body clenches. The wren of anxiety flies down my throat and circles in my stomach, flapping her wings.

"Let's go," Dad says, picking up a bottle carrier containing empty lemon squash bottles. Mum had filled them with fizzy water from the SodaStream for me.

Sitting in the car on the motorway, we don't speak to each other. We're only just back from a wonderful trip to Lavenham where we stayed in the historic Swan Hotel, and I saw Mary and met her new dog.

Yesterday afternoon I was celebrating with a male friend that my book will soon be published. I leave my cat for two days and this happens. My chest is crushed with the worst pain I have ever felt. This is worse than when my grandfathers died, worse than when Seb split up with me. I can't understand why G-d would take away my life-saving kitten.

"Mum?" I call, sliding open the front door.

"Sweetie," Mum says, her eyes red from crying. "I couldn't sleep last night, worrying about my precious angel."

She looks so drained, I put my arm around her. "Maybe he got locked in someone's garage or …"

"The neighbours have all checked their sheds and garages." Mum says.

We have a WhatsApp group in the Warren which was set up at the beginning of lockdown.

"Maybe someone has stolen him because he looks so valuable." I say. He has long orange fur with a huge ruff round his neck and a long fluffy tail. There are darker orange stripes on the top of his head.

The house feels his loss, it's so quiet and still without him. I post on Facebook asking everyone to check their garages and sheds. Mum puts a post on Nextdoor and makes an advert for Instagram which flashes up frequently. There are no sightings.

I try to focus on publicity for *In Bloom* but the PTSD I felt when Seb split up with me has come back. I can't even look at a pack of tarot cards. Every day Mum tramps the streets for hours, calling his name. I post him in a missing pets Facebook group.

My aunty and uncle make some laminated posters of him which Mum puts up as far as Shenley in all our local roads, and kind friends put them up in Borehamwood.

There continue to be no sightings. I still think he has been stolen. My heart is utterly broken, and I can't stop crying.

"We just have to hope that, wherever he is, he is being looked after." Mum says as we sit on the grey sofa: unable to read, unable even to watch television.

"If he had been run over and taken to a vet, they would have scanned his microchip." I say.

"I have been to all the local vets, and they all have posters of him, he must be alive." Mum says, sipping her glass of Sauvignon.

"I want him back," I say. "Why is G-d doing this to us?"

"I don't know sweetie," Mum says, putting her arm around me. We cry on each other's shoulders.

"I think I've found your cat," a girl's voice says on the other end of the line.

"He's orange and fluffy and very big. I've got him inside now."

"We're coming," Mum says. "Come on darling." It's 8.10 p.m. and we jump into the car and drive to the other end of Radlett.

When we park outside the block of flats, we see a girl standing in the doorway. "We're looking for our cat," Mum says.

"Here he is," she says, opening the door and shutting it behind us as we go in. In the hallway is a large, pale orange cat.

"Thank you so much for trying to help, but that is not our cat." Mum says. She is holding back her tears; I can hear it in her voice.

"What a beautiful cat." I say.

"He shouldn't be out at night so near the main road." Mum says. He just sits there.

"I think I know where he lives," Mum says. "Let's put him in the basket and take him home." She holds open the door of Fluffball's carrier but the cat won't go inside. He dashes off into the night and sits by the row of cars parked at the front of the block, just by the main road.

"Thank you again," Mum says to the girl. "I'm going to talk to his owner now."

Deflated, we drag ourselves back to the car. Crossing the main road, we take the first left and stop a few houses down. Mum goes up to the door. She returns, ashen-faced, a few moments later.

"That woman was so rude to me, I just don't understand it." Mum says.

"I said I'd found her cat and that she ought to keep him in at night rather than letting him cross the busy main road, but she screamed at me and told me to keep my nose out of her business."

"He could have been killed," I say as we drive home.

"No one has ever been that rude to me before," Mum says, clenching her hands on the steering wheel, her knuckles white. "I was trying to help her."

Another week goes by. I still can't look at my tarot cards. I'm sleeping 'til nine thirty in the morning, only stirring when Mum wakes me. Our lives have shrunk anyway during the pandemic of course, but now, all we do is look for our cat.

Every afternoon Mum traipses the streets, rain or shine. Sometimes a kind friend keeps her company. Everyone in Radlett knows Fluffball as he has such a large territory and is so bold and friendly. All our neighbours are looking for him. It's October so the weather is getting colder. The evenings are the worst, when Fluffball should be curled up on the sofa next to us, but isn't.

My heart is smashed to a pulp. I pray to G-d to bring my cat back, but he is not listening. And yet, we are convinced he's not dead or someone would've told us.

Round and round in circles. Has he been stolen? Perhaps he's happy with a new family. He must be out of the area as there are no sightings apart from people mistaking one of the three Maine coons at the other end of the village for him – one of whom we've just encountered.

We are never going to see our precious angel again. Never going to kiss his stripy head or hear his chirrup for food or his loud miaow when he comes in. This is Rock Bottom, I know. This is the worst thing that has happened in my life and it's up against serious competition.

Chapter 45

"Spitfire has been found," Dad says, as I enter the living room after my afternoon sleep.

I look at Dad: "Where?"

"He's up a tree," Dad says. "Five doors down the road at the bottom of a neighbour's garden. Mum is down there with him, trying to coax him down."

"Are you sure?" I ask, unable to take this in.

"Someone on the Warren WhatsApp group just put up a message saying 'There's a cat in my tree,' with a picture of him. Several people messaged back saying 'That's Spitfire.'"

I rush into the hall and put on my coat. It's early November, Bonfire Night in fact, almost three weeks since he went missing.

"I'm going to investigate," I say, opening the front door. Walking as fast as I can down the road, I turn down the side of the fifth house along. Walking to the bottom of the garden, I see Mum with a blanket round her shoulders.

I hear his piteous cries before I see him. Looking up, I see my cat in an enormous oak tree with no lower branches. It's impossible for him to get down, it's too far, and on one side of the tree there's a huge drop to a tennis court. I can't imagine why he climbed so far up – he's about thirty feet from the ground. He must have been chased by something.

"Mum," I say.

"Sweetie," Mum says, smiling and putting her arms around me, first putting down the tin of tuna which our kind neighbour brought to try to coax him down.

"How long have you been here?" I ask. Above us our cat is calling to us. His cries pull at my heart strings.

"I saw the message at about half past one on the WhatsApp group," Mum says, her voice shaking. "I've been here since then trying to persuade him to start coming down but he is too frightened. An electrician working nearby came with an extendible ladder, climbed the tree and caught Fluffball. He had him under one arm, but the poor little thing struggled free and climbed further up the tree."

"Oh no," I say, looking up at my precious angel who is crying for us.

"As soon as he saw me, he started crying," Mum says. "Our neighbour rang the RSPCA and they said they wouldn't come as it wasn't an emergency. They said if a cat can get up a tree it can get down – not our Fluffball. The fire brigade also refused to help."

"But it is an emergency." I say. He could die up there. We wait at the bottom of the tree and after about half an hour Fluffball descends to a point which is within reach of the ladder. The brave electrician is willing to have another go.

"Be careful," Mum says.

He makes it up to the top of the huge ladder, just above the fork in the branches where Spitfire is sitting, reaches out his arms and pulls Spitfire towards him. The poor terrified cat struggles but the amazing man tucks him under one arm and climbs down the ladder. Time slows down, at every step we wait with bated breath for Spitfire to struggle free, but somehow, they reach the ground together.

"Here you go," he says, handing Spitfire to Mum. He's a big chap with a kind face.

"Thank you so much," Mum says. "I could never thank you enough. There's nothing of you, my precious," she says to Spitfire. I put a hand out to stroke him. He seems very weak and very still.

"Let's get you home," Mum says, and we begin the short walk home.

"So, apparently," Mum says once we've got Spitfire safely inside. "He's been pulling out his fur to make a nest. The electrician said there was a pile of fur in the fork of the tree and also some evidence of toilet activity. He must have been up there the whole time."

"Poor baby," I say sitting next to him.

"It's lucky it rained such a lot," Mum says. "He must have been surviving on rainwater all this time."

"Do you think he was up the tree for nearly three weeks?" I say, gazing at the stripy head I thought I was never going to see again.

"Yes," Mum says. "And it's only now the leaves have died and fallen that he became visible."

"He could have died up there." I say, stroking him under his chin. He purrs: a tiny engine rumbling.

"I'm just going to phone the vet," Mum says.

"Hello, oh hi Louisa, we've found Spitfire." Mum says over the phone. Louisa is Spitfire's favourite vet.

"He was trapped up a tree, yes, of course I'll bring him in tomorrow." She puts the phone down. Spitfire crunches through a small amount of his dried food.

"Louisa says we should feed him very small meals as there is a danger of him suffering from refeeding syndrome after so long without food."

Spitfire cuddles up with me on my furry blanket. I photograph him and post on Facebook "We've found Spitfire." The whole of Radlett rejoices that he is home.

At nine thirty the next morning Mum comes into my room to wake me. "I'm taking Fluffball to the vet now," she says.

I spend the morning doing my barre class and posting "Spitfire has been found," on all the lost pets Facebook groups.

"Spitfire has lost nearly one and a half kilos," Mum says on her return from the vet. "Louisa says we have to keep him inside for two weeks and feed him little and often to build up his strength. She has taken some blood to check his liver and kidney function and I have to take him back next week."

"Poor Fluffball," I say. "He won't like staying in."

"It's lucky he was a little overweight," Mum says, "or he could have died."

Fluffball, however, was quite happy to stay in as he was very weak and tired and his blood tests revealed that his liver and kidneys were not working very well. He was not very hungry at first and just wanted to sleep all the time, but he did get used to a little snack in the early hours of the morning and has not wanted to give that up. Gradually, he began to seem more like his own self and his next lot of blood tests showed a significant improvement. After two weeks we let him go outside for a short time each day, but we were on tenterhooks till he came home.

I expect to feel better now Spitfire's home, but I don't. The panther isn't here but I'm Not Quite Right. I continue sleeping until Mum wakes me at nine thirty each morning and I go to bed at 9 p.m. each night.

The wren of anxiety flutters around my stomach, beating her wings.

"How are we ever going to stop worrying about him when he goes out?" I ask Mum as we sit in Fluffball's room. He is eating his supper.

"We will gradually learn to trust him again," Mum says. "He didn't run away on purpose, he just climbed a tree and couldn't get down. We have seen him do that in the garden, but we have always been able to help him down. This was a much taller tree."

"But why did he run up that tree in the first place?" I wonder, listening to Spitfire slurping the juice from his food. I can see his ribs.

"Perhaps a fox or a dog chased him," Mum says. "All the time I was traipsing the streets calling for him it's possible he could hear me."

"Don't torture yourself Mum," I say, putting my arms round her. "He's home now, we are so lucky to have him back."

"I thought I'd never see that stripy head again," Mum says.

"I know," I say. "I thought the same."

We look at our silly Fluffball as he stretches after his meal and begins the arduous process of cleaning himself, beginning with licking his tail.

Thank you G-d, for returning my life-saving kitten to me, I think.

Chapter 46

Lockdown is hard for everyone, it goes without saying. Family members in different parts of the country not being allowed to visit each other. People on their own, having no one with whom to form a bubble.

However, in one way it's particularly difficult for me. As the months stretch on, I am unable to write anything good, unable since October the eighteenth to look at my tarot cards. I know that time out of my precious short life is being stolen from me.

My health deteriorates during lockdown. At the beginning I can barre standing up, but by March of 2021 I can merely lie on the floor to exercise, due to the pain in my back that I now know is cancer.

My brilliant teacher continues to put on classes six times a week and we become good friends. It's barre on Monday and Wednesday, Pilates on Tuesday, Friday and Saturday and personal training on Thursday.

We have a few minutes to chat before the class and sometimes up to twenty minutes after. Our little group grows closer. There are six of us including our teacher. After lockdown is over, the barre crew start coming to visit me in my garden.

But, for six months after Fluffball goes missing, I can't even look at my tarot cards. I'm flooded with anxiety, each time he leaves the house, that he won't come back. My thoughts return, obsessively, to him up a tree in the dark and rain being cold, hungry and frightened.

I don't know how much he remembers but his behaviour changes. He stays close to the house and pops in several times during the morning for extra breakfasts. He used to stay out for much longer periods of time, although he has never been allowed out at night.

In March his hay fever returns. He is probably allergic to tree pollen. We are usually able to control it with steroids and they work for a while, but in April he starts scratching below his eye and makes a hole in his face. Mum takes him to the vet who puts him on Piriton and advises keeping him inside for a week. Poor Fluffball, he doesn't understand and paces around the house looking defeated and miserable. However, after less than a week, his eyes have stopped streaming and his face is starting to heal. We decide to let him out again and, so far, the Piriton and steroids have done the trick. He now stays out from about seven thirty in the morning till about five in the afternoon, with several visits home for extra snacks.

People who say, "Cats are no trouble," haven't met my Spitfire – he's in the hospital almost as often as I am. However, he seems to know how ill I am, lying on my bed for hours with me when I can't get up.

Recently, Mum has been sitting with me whilst I have my bath, and Spitfire comes in too, putting his front paws up on the edge of the bath, sometimes jumping up so he can stand on the edge as he used to do when he was a kitten.

He's so precious, my angel Fluffball. I thank G-d every day for bringing him back to me.

As suddenly as my mood had dropped, it comes up again, mid-March.

A barre friend has a tarot reading: I can look at my cards again. Then another barre friend. She introduces me to her chum who asks for a reading for her daughter. The daughter is so impressed she buys readings for two other people.

Through March I do twenty-three readings and earn a respectable amount of money, doing something I love and am good at. I adore the regimented nature of the tarot: learning the meanings of the cards, reading books about their history. It's a system combining astrology, hermeticism and Kabbalah. I try to keep my readings as positive as possible as we have free will to achieve the optimum future for ourselves. News of my talent spreads like wildfire by word of mouth and I'm so happy that at last, aged almost forty-two, I've found work I can do whilst lying in bed.

Last term, January till March, I did an amazing astrology course taught by Richard Swatton called Symbolic Doorways which was about training, intuition, the aura, dreams, spirit and how to place astrology in the esoteric, hermetic tradition. This has really helped me to rely more on my intuition whilst doing tarot, as has Brigit Esselmont's *Intuitive Tarot*. I know the cards well enough now to write their basic meanings but also to communicate my feelings about what I see in the cards.

And my customers are impressed: people come back for repeat readings, recommend me to friends, who in turn recommend me to others. I try to use as much astrology in my tarot as I can because the two disciplines are so entwined. I always have a tarot or astrology book on the go.

I've just read Mary Greer's *The Meaning of the Tarot Court Cards*" and I have cleared shelves in my old playroom to house all my new tarot and astrology books.

As my physical health deteriorates, I'm more determined than ever to keep my brain working. Let's just hope I will be well enough soon to return to chemotherapy as I really don't want the cancer to reach my skull and brain.

There are so many books left to read. I've just read the brilliant Susan Howatch Starbridge novels, about the state of the Church of England in the twentieth century, and I've ordered the whole Blandings series by P.G. Wodehouse for a little light reading. I already have *Heavy Weather* and it's wonderfully funny. Recently I've only been reading other memoirs and books on astrology and tarot: I need a break to read for pleasure.

Chapter 47

Exercise for Mental Health

Exercise saves my life and I do it every day. But, if you're not in a good exercise regime and need a push, here are some tips:

- Find a form of exercise you love and do it every day. It genuinely doesn't matter what. Are you an outdoors person? If so, running, walking and cycling are the ones for you. There's a trend towards wild swimming at the moment which strikes me as Too Cold, but swimming in a heated pool uses every muscle in your body. I love swimming on holiday in an outdoor pool or in the sea where it is warm when you get out.

- If you're going to join a gym, make sure it's walking distance from home or a short drive. If it is too far out of your way you won't go. When I was living in my flat, I was a ten-minute walk from Virgin Active in Cricklewood so I would walk there and do my grocery shopping on the way home.

- Throughout lockdown, Zoom exercise classes have really taken off, so if you want to do Pilates, barre or aerobics, for example, they are available at the touch of a button. You may need basic equipment such as a stretchy band, booty band, a small or large ball, and light hand weights. My Zoom barre and Pilates are a godsend.

- Leg weights will enhance the effectiveness of your walking.
- Exercise with a friend. Mum has walked all through lockdown with her friends. You're catching up and seeing the countryside: it's a win/win situation.
- If you have an exercise bike, get onto Peloton or an online cycling class. Or head back to the Spin studio now lockdown is over.
- Join Borrow My Doggy for the best walking companion – a canine one. Or borrow a friend's dog for an hour or go walking with a friend and their dog. This makes walking a social activity.
- If you're lucky enough to have a dog, do canicross. You need a special harness which goes round the dog and clips to your belt, so you can run safely attached to your dog.
- If you're out of practice, buy a few sessions with a personal trainer. You'll work harder and more effectively. You can do this in your garden, in a studio or at home.
- Mum has a Fitbit and brother has a Garmin. Get one and aim for 10,000 steps per day.
- Charities run challenges all the time. I have a friend walking 100,000 steps in a month to raise money for refugees and my Pilates teacher just raised £4,000 by running 1,000 kilometres in a month for Breast Cancer Care.
- Be open to trying new things. You may find you hate rock climbing or surfing but try activities you haven't experienced before.
- What time of day are you at your best? I'm a morning person so I do classes then. You may be a night owl, in which case an evening class would suit you.
- The most important thing is to schedule time for exercise in your diary. Make it an appointment you don't break, for example straight after dropping your children at school, or in your lunch break or after supper. If it's written down, you'll be more likely to do it.

- If you're dieting, this is an added incentive to schedule some exercise into your day, as then you'll be able to consume more calories. But of course, make sure there's still a calorie deficit.
- Gardening is exercise, as is cleaning.
- Always take the stairs rather than a lift or escalator. But you can always walk up or down an escalator.
- Make it fun: purchase some workout gear you love so you can feel good whilst toning up. There's a new shop in Radlett which stocks designer exercise clothes, but I also recommend Sweaty Betty and Victoria's Secret.
- Buy a course of riding lessons. This may lead to a life-long love of horses and eventually your own horse, or it may not. I rode regularly from the ages of five to eighteen and always try to ride on holiday.

Chapter 48

How does it feel to know your death is imminent? The first thing: now I will do anything to stay alive. It may not look pretty as I toss and turn and sweat in Mum's bed, kicking her, delirious with a chemo-induced fever, or as I kneel at the loo puking my guts out. But that's my reality.

The first chemo we try in this new round of palliative treatment is eribulin. It gives me a high temperature two days after the infusion. Mum phones the hospital and the nurses tell her to take me to A & E as there is a danger I might have developed sepsis. My parents and I clamber into the Mercedes at eight o'clock at night, Dad driving. They admit me at Watford and my parents are not allowed to accompany me, although they are my carers, because of Covid. Sweating, I lie in bed in a ward. Doctors give me antibiotics for the possible sepsis. During the night I toss and turn. In the morning my temperature has dropped but it is up again by the next evening.

The doctors don't seem to know what is wrong with me. I lie in my bed on a ward surrounded by the sick and dying.

I don't mind the hustle and bustle of the ward and feel quite safe with the nurses' station in the middle of the room, beds in rows up against two walls. They let me go two days later, having been unable to ascertain whether or not I have an infection. I don't of course. My parents and I are convinced it is all side effects of the chemo.

"You're home, darling." Mums says, wrapping her arms around me. "My precious, how do you feel?"

"OK," I say. "Where's Fluffball?"

"He's on his chair in the library," Mum says. The library used to be our old playroom. The walls are lined with books: memoirs, novels, books on history and travel, biographies and all my astrology and tarot reading material.

"I'm going back to bed," I say and lie there all day. My temperature returns in the evening and Mum decides I had better sleep with her so she can feed me paracetamol during the night. She carries my hypoallergenic pillows up to her room and Dad is demoted to my brother's room.

I toss and turn during the night and sweat all over Mum, but wake up at six in the morning, bright and cheerful and temperature down. I decide to go back to my own bed, taking my smoky quartz point for sleep and my green calcite for reducing temperature. I walk slowly down the stairs with my pillows under one arm.

Back in bed, I lie down, weak but still alive. This pattern continues for the next month of treatment: one more visit to A & E where they give me medication for possible sepsis, then my week off, then another three-night stretch of fever at night monitored by Mum.

"You kicked me in the night," Mum says.

"I'm sorry, I didn't mean to," I say. Fluffball gazes at me from the floor.

"We're so lucky to have our precious angel back," I say to Mum, stroking him under his chin. He purrs.

"I don't know how we'd keep going without him," Mum says, gazing at me with her eyes full of pity.

"Why are you looking at me like that?" I ask her.

"Because you look so fragile," she says. "Believe me, if I could take this pain away from you, I would."

"Don't be silly," I say. "I need you. Dad and Carl and Fluffball need you."

Fluffball climbs onto the bed next to me and stretches diagonally across it. There is no room for anyone else with six kilograms of cat spread out in an arrow from bottom left to top right.

"Good morning Fluffball," I say, kissing the stripy top of his head. "Thank G-d you came back."

"He's your little fluffy nurse," Mum says, and it's true. Since this latest episode of illness he wants to be with me all the time, having my afternoon sleep with me, sitting on my bed whilst I do tarot. One day, I stumble into bed for my afternoon sleep and he stretches out next to me under the covers. We sleep together.

When I wake up, he tries and fails to make his way out from under the covers. I lift them up in the end so he can jump down to the floor. It's six p.m., we've been sleeping since just after lunch.

"Supper, Fluffball," I say, and he trots up to his bedroom. Following him, I find Mum in the kitchen.

"Fluffball would like his supper now," I say. Mum takes the packet of wet food from the fridge: he has wet food for breakfast and supper with dried food several times during the day and once in the middle of the night. Fluffball turns his head and chirrups to make sure we are following him as he thumps up the stairs and into his room. He sits by his bowl and, as Mum squeezes out the food, he licks the juice from the packet.

"Fluffball won't let me die," I say. He's my life-saving kitten: obtained six months after my breast cancer diagnosis in 2013, six months after the death of our previous cat Romario, who we always called Furry. We love him beyond words, beyond articulation, beyond everything. The time during which he was missing was the worst three weeks of my life.

"We'd better do a scan," the oncologist says as we sit in his office. "Let's see if a month of eribulin has helped you."

"OK," I say, thinking it must have done after all those terrible side effects.

"Ring up Bushey and I'll organise a scan," he says. "You look well."

"Thank you," I say. I don't want to keep going to A & E, could you arrange for me to be admitted to Bushey after my next treatment?"

"I'll see what I can do," he says, scribbling in his notes.

And so, straight after my next chemo, I'm admitted to the hospital where I am a frequent inpatient. They dose me up with paracetamol and I don't develop a temperature. It's a bit of respite for my parents who, due to Covid restrictions, are not allowed to visit me.

Eating the lovely hospital food, not being ill, watching television sitting up in my comfortable hospital bed, I'm content. I will see my parentals and my Fluffball soon, but in the meantime, I sleep well and eat well.

After three days with no temperature, I go home to wait for my scan the following week: my week off chemo. Things don't seem so bad as I lie in bed reading *Tarot and Astrology*. *The chemo must be working*, I tell myself.

Chapter 49

"I'm afraid the scan is not good," my oncologist says. "There are new spots on your bones and in your liver."

We're sitting in his office. Behind him it is sunny, but the trees are still bare. It's early spring.

"What are we going to do?" I ask, crying. The nurse puts her arms around me. "Sorry, it's a bit of a shock."

"We're going to try something else," he says. There's a new drug combination a few of my patients are on."

"How are they tolerating it?" I ask.

"Well." He always says this about everything, including the capecitabine which caused all the skin to come off my feet, and I felt as if I had been hit by a train by about eleven each morning.

"I suppose I had better try it." I say. "What is it called?"

"It's called GemCarbo – gemcitabine and carboplatin. The first week is both drugs, the second week just gemcitabine and then a week off. We'll start on Monday."

"OK," I say, feeling shocked. I can't believe the last chemo has not only failed to work but has also enabled the cancer to spread.

"I'll see you on Monday," he says. "I'll pop in to see how you are doing."

"Thank you," I say. I'm on my own, Dad isn't allowed to be with me. I start crying again.

"There, there," the nurse says, putting her arms around me. I cry on her shoulder out of despair and exhaustion. How can the chemo have failed to work when it has made me so ill? I can't believe it. And yet, it's true.

"GemCarbo is good," she says. "We have several people on it. You'll be fine."

"I hope so," I say sniffing, thinking about my cancerous liver and the cancer spreading in my bones.

"On the plus side," the oncologist says, "It hasn't reached your skull or brain."

"I'm glad about that," I say. "Sorry for making a fuss."

"You're not making a fuss," the nurse says. "You're upset. But GemCarbo is going to work, sweetie."

I put my sweater on and take a deep breath, wiping my eyes, blowing my nose.

"What happened?" Dad asks when I return to the car.

"The chemo isn't working," I say, gazing out of the windscreen at the hedge, spotting the white scut of a rabbit disappearing into the hedge.

"There's new cancer in my bones and liver but not yet, thank G-d, in my skull or brain."

"Well, that's something," Dad says, pragmatic as always.

"I start GemCarbo on Monday," I say. "I've got a leaflet about it in my bag."

"We'll look at it when we get home," Dad says. "I'm sure your doctor knows what he's doing."

"I cried," I say. "I cried on the nurse."

"That's fine," Dad says. "We'll look at the leaflet with Mum when we get home."

Gazing out of the window, I see the shut-down pub and then a field of horses. The branches are still bare but soon it will be spring. And I wish to be alive for the spring – my favourite time of year: the clay court tennis season, artichokes, English asparagus, the arrival of the house martins from Africa in late April, my birthday in May.

At home, Mum is waiting up by the front door, doing *The Times* crossword, Fluffball sitting next to her on the sofa. She starts as she sees us and opens the door.

"The chemo isn't working," I say, "So I'm starting GemCarbo on Monday.

"What's that?" Mum asks. "How can the drug not be working? It's made you so ill."

"It's not doing anything," I say. "There is new cancer in my liver, there are more spots on my bones."

"My poor darling," Mum says, putting her arms around me. I just cry and cry.

By Monday, after barre and a chat with my exercise chums, I'm ready for GemCarbo. Side effects seem similar to eribulin, according to the leaflet, but no hair loss, so every cloud has a silver lining: maybe my hair will grow back a little.

At the hospital, Luisa makes me a bed by flattening my chair and putting a sheet underneath me, a pillow for my head and blanket over me. She is my favourite nurse. First the saline solution to flush my port, then the carboplatin and finally the gemcitabine. I lie there, exhausted, drifting in and out of consciousness as she changes the bag of fluid.

"It work, this one," she says. She's from Spain.

"I hope it works," I say.

"It good drug, we have many people on it." She smiles at me. She has lots of freckles, a button nose, big brown eyes and curly dark brown hair.

"How are the children?" I ask. They are five and two and run her ragged.

"They good, little terrors," she says, laughing. "They exhausts me, work is hard but they are harder."

"I hope they like this," I say, giving her some Easter chocolate with pictures of chicks and eggs on it.

"So kind of you, thank you," she says with a chuckle. "I eat this myself."

After about three hours, I'm done.

"See you on Friday for bloods," she says.

"Bye everyone, see you on Friday," I say. Walking out to the car, I feel a new sense of hope that this treatment will work, and I will have a spring and summer. Due to Covid there will be no spectators at the tennis tournaments in Monte Carlo, Barcelona and Madrid but there may be some at the big one for us Rafaholics – Roland-Garros. I will be alive for it.

I love Rafa because of how determined he is, how he fights for every point as if it's match point, how he's constantly looking for new ways to improve. He's my inspiration and surely, along with Roger Federer, the Greatest of All Time.

"How was it?" Dad asks. He's picking me up as Mum is playing bridge online.

"Good," I say, "It's going to work and I'm going to have spring and summer."

"Yes, of course you are," Dad says. Driving out of the hospital grounds, we see two rabbits munching on the grass at the top of the hill.

Chapter 50

How to be Happy

- What does happiness mean to you? Write it down, see what is missing from your life and try to build it in. With happiness, like with everything else, there must be an abundance mindset. You probably already have most of what you feel you need.

- Find pleasure in small things. For example, I would love a dog more than anything in the world, but I can have dog friends, such as Gandalf the liver flat-coated retriever. Now that I am too ill to take him for a walk for an hour, I see him less. His owners sometimes bring him round to visit me so I can cuddle him and give him treats.

- Get a pet. They reduce loneliness, anxiety, stress and frustration. My precious angel Spitfire is such an amazing nurse to me: sitting on my bed next to me, purring. He goes out about seven thirty in the morning after breakfast and comes in for lunch after a busy morning patrolling his territory. After lunch he wanders very slowly to the hedge at the front of our garden under which he sits until Mum calls him in the late afternoon. He is very good and when he is called he comes trotting down the road.

- Write a gratitude list each morning. I'm lucky to be easily pleased: watching the birds in the garden always makes me feel better. I see the wood pigeons chasing the magpies, the blue tits and great tits coming to blows over the fat balls. Today I saw robins courting, I hope they will soon be rearing chicks. The soap opera of their lives is so absorbing.

- Put things you want onto your Amazon wish list so if anyone wants to buy you a present, you can show them your list.

- Whenever you can, take advantage of free gifts. PayPal has a new service where you can purchase an item and spread the payment over six months.

- Write everything you spend in a book. I have a midnight blue, crushed velvet covered notebook in which I write my income and expenditure. This really helps me see how much I'm earning from tarot reading and how much money I'm putting back into my business. My tarot deck collection and astrology course accounts for most of the money I spend. Of course, tarot and astrology interpretations are changing all the time so I have to keep buying new books to keep up.

- Check your bank account every day to make sure you know how much you are spending. This is particularly important as I have had fraud on my card a few times, so I need to know when this happens.

- Talk to a friend. A problem shared is a problem solved or, if not solved, at least ameliorated. I try to speak to my best friends every day. I exchange messages with my brother in Abroad every day, and we speak about three times a week.

- Exercise – find something you enjoy and go for it. See the chapter on Exercise for Mental Health.

- Write every day, whether or not you feel like it. It will become a habit. Try doing morning pages: when you wake up, before reading a book or a newspaper or listening to the radio, put pen to paper and write whatever comes into your head. This is automatic writing. You get into a flow state – a stream of consciousness – if you do this every morning for ten, fifteen, or more minutes. I'm writing about eight A4 pages per day, double spaced, at the moment, as the end of my deadline approaches. The Sword of Damocles is hanging over my head. Soon my head will be severed from my body as I write, write, write.

- Find a job or hobby you enjoy so much that you become engrossed in it. I find this with reading, writing, exercise, astrology and tarot.
- Visit wildlife centres, parks, zoos and safari parks. At London Zoo, where I used to work, I wander around the whole zoo chatting to the volunteers. I need to make it to the zoo soon to see the new Sumatran tiger.
- Ride or cycle: exercise by sitting down. When my parents were first dating Dad learnt to ride a horse as Mum loved it so much.
- Be in the moment. Live every day as if it's the last day of your life. What would your dream day contain? What time would you wake up? Try waking up an hour earlier to have a wash, write, pull a tarot card for the day, and check your horoscope. I'm a Taurus sun, Capricorn moon and Libra rising. Sun: character. Moon: behaviour. Rising/ascendant: how you come across. Study. Learn new things each day, week, month or year. Before I started my astrology course I did short courses on a variety of topics: advanced tarot, equine behaviour, feline psychology, Jungian dream analysis and farm management. Also, two courses through the Paranormal Academy – witchcraft and wicca, and mythical and legendary animals. I love to learn new information about whatever subject I choose. I loved school and have always been happy in a classroom. Be enthusiastic about each new subject, variety is the spice of life.
- Volunteer if you can. I volunteered at London Zoo and at Waverley Carriage Driving for the Disabled. I got so much

pleasure from my voluntary work. If you're doing something to help others, the volunteer managers will be pleased with you as will the clients. You will feel the warm glow of helpfulness.

- Hug people. It's been really tough not being able to hug my friends or anyone except my parents during Covid. Couldn't even hug brother until he'd been here for twelve days which was sad.

- Make a bucket list of places to visit before you die (although I'm not sure how much travelling will be happening in this Covid world). I had always wanted to go to Venice. Mum said I'd have to wait for my husband to take me. However, by the age of thirty-eight I had no husband, so Mum and I went to Venice together. It was magical. I would love to go on more river cruises like the Danube one we went on just after a particularly unpleasant course of chemotherapy with capecitabine. My feet were covered with huge blisters and I could hardly walk but I recovered enough to enjoy the outings as we cruised through Austria, Hungary, Serbia and Croatia, past the beautiful riverside scenery. I'd still love to visit Malta, the Brontë House, the ospreys at Lake Garten, as well as Australia, New Zealand and Madagascar. Unfortunately, I'm not well enough for long-haul flights.

- Take up knitting. You can do it anywhere – in front of the television, in bed, on a train. It's uniquely portable and mess-free for a craft. I've made scarves for many people, and at the moment I am doing one for my cousin's new baby.

- Find a television show you love and watch it. A few months ago, we watched season four of *The Crown* and then, because Mum hadn't seen them, we watched the first three seasons.

- Write cards to people you love. They will really appreciate the gesture.

- Smile. Fake it till you make it. Talk to everyone. People love to talk and be listened to.

Chapter 51

APRIL 2021

I'm kneeling in front of the loo puking my guts out. I feel terrible. It's two days after my last chemo. I've coped with it well so far but now I can't stop being sick. G-d knows how long I've been kneeling here. Time stands still as I heave and yet more brown vomit comes up. I also have diarrhoea and feel dizzy. My legs are weak, I must have a temperature.

"Darling, what are you doing in there?" Mum's voice breaks into my brittle mind.

"Being sick," I shout back. I don't want to open the door and let her in.

"Come out of there," Mum says as another stream of vomit bursts up and out. I sit on the loo feeling another bout of diarrhoea approaching, dropping my head to try to stop feeling sick but it doesn't work.

Eventually I make it out of the bathroom. Collapsing on the sofa, I close my eyes.

"Let's take your temperature," Mum says, brandishing the thermometer and looking at me with pity and concern. My temperature is 38.9 degrees which is high. It's Wednesday. By Friday the constant nausea has eased.

On Saturday night Passover begins with the Seder. We join some friends on Zoom and I wear my new dark green dress. I notice that, despite all the weight I've lost, it is tight on my arms and stomach. I manage to stay awake for a little while, then exhaustion forces me back to bed.

The next day, in the bath, I notice that my legs are shiny and swollen.

"Right, I'm taking you to the hospital," Mum says.

At the cancer hospital they take some blood. I'm exhausted. We go home and arrange to come back in the afternoon. When we return, Mum is allowed in with me for once. My oncologist comes to see me.

"Cordelia," he says in a concerned voice. "Your platelet level has dropped to two, it should be about one hundred and fifty, you must go straight to A & E, you need urgent medical attention. Take this letter with you."

"I'll put a gripper in your port so they can get fluids in and out of you," Luisa says. "Wait, sharp scratch, the gripper is in." Sue tapes it up. It's almost five o'clock.

"We've got to go to A & E," I say to Mum.

"OK, darling," she says.

"My legs and arms are swollen," I say to Luisa. "I don't know why that should be," she says. I lie collapsed in my chair, I'm so tired.

We go home and I pack a bag: tarot cards, a few pairs of knickers and socks, a couple of sleepwear tops. At A & E my parents drop me at reception, they are not allowed in with me. I produce the letter from my oncologist and, although Luisa had phoned to tell them to expect me, the receptionist claims to know nothing about me.

I sit in A & E with my bag on my lap. There's a chap wearing a rugby shirt with blood all over his face opposite me. Eventually I'm taken to a room and left there, someone brings me an egg sandwich which I eat as I am so hungry, even though it is Passover and I shouldn't be eating bread. After some time, a doctor arrives.

"Let's get some blood out of your port," he says. He fiddles with it but can't make it work.

"I know it works," I say. "They have just attached the gripper at the cancer hospital."

"I'll find someone to help," he says and disappears. Left on my own I go onto Amazon and buy a fluorescent pink wig for £10.99.

A pair of doctors come in, they also cannot work the port and go away again. The bright lighting in the room prevents me falling asleep, even though I'm desperately tired.

Another doctor arrives, "We're going to put a cannula in your foot," he says after yet another attempt to get the port to work.

"You won't be able to get any blood out of my foot," I say, remembering the last time a doctor tried this and how painful and unsuccessful it was.

"We have to," he says.

"I'm going home," I say, picking up my bag, pulling on my wig and trousers.

"You can't," he says.

"I'm going to," I say. "I'm discharging myself. It's disgraceful that not one of five doctors can work my port."

I get up and walk to the doctors' station, it's nine in the evening now and I need to go home.

"I have to go, I'm discharging myself," I say to one of the doctors.

"Are you sure that's a good idea?" he asks, eyes full of concern.

"I'm sure." I say.

"Fill in this discharge form," he says, so I do and having signed it I go out of A & E. Sitting on the wall outside, I can see the full moon. I call my parents.

"What's going on?" Mum asks.

"I've just discharged myself from hospital," I say. "Five doctors couldn't work my port. Please come and get me."

"But it's nine o'clock," Mum says.

"I just need a good night's sleep in my own bed. We'll go back to the cancer hospital in the morning."

"OK, we're on our way," Mum says.

Twenty minutes later the Mercedes draws up and I crawl in. My phone rings, it's my brother.

"Luisa just called to see what was going on. I told her, and she said you must stay in the hospital. There's a risk you could bleed to death internally if you don't get some platelets this evening."

"I can't," I say. "Five doctors couldn't work my port. I need to sleep in my own bed. I'm not going to die tonight."

"I'll call and tell her," my brother says.

Soon we are home and I take my night-time meds and fall asleep.

The next day, when I wake up, we go back to the cancer hospital. Luisa attaches a syringe to my port, and I see the blood flow out.

"It work," she says.

"Of course it does," I say. "I'm never going back to A & E."

"We will give you a platelet transfusion here," she says, "And then you will be admitted to Spire for a few days for some more transfusions. Your oncologist is away now but another doctor will look after you there."

"Phew," I say, flooded with relief. I have my bag with me and I'm not wearing a wig. I look skeletal, like death. Not even warmed up. Cold death. The platelets are yellow, they look like pressed apple juice. I close my eyes, exhausted, as they flood in.

At Spire hospital I get into bed. The doctor comes to see me. He is a lovely, kind, gentle man. I find out later that he is a geriatrician.

"Hi, I'm Doctor Goldberg," he says. "We need to get some blood into you, one bag now and another this evening. What do you think?"

His voice is gentle. "Yes please, thank you," I say.

"I'll go and arrange the blood transfusion," he says.

"I'm just so tired," I say, my eyes drifting shut.

"You just stay where you are and rest," he says, looking at me with his soft brown eyes.

"Thank you," I say. He turns out the light and I doze. It's still morning and I'm probably not going to sleep but … there's a knock on my door which jolts me from my slumber.

"Here we are," my doctor says, carrying a bag of bright red fluid. "If you don't mind just sitting up, there's a good girl."

He hooks the bag onto a metal stand and wheels it over to me. "So, this should take about four hours," he says.

"There's a gripper in my port which the nurses put in at Elstree." I say.

"Excellent," he says, smiling at me with those liquid brown eyes.

I take the tape off the port, and he flushes it with saline.

"All set," he says, as he feeds the plastic tube from the bag into the dangling plastic tube on the end of my port. I see the bright red blood flowing in. "I'll come and check on you later."

"See you later," I say.

"We'll get you sorted out," he says, conviction in his soft voice.

I close my eyes and fall asleep.

About thirty minutes later there's a knock on my door.

"What would you like for lunch and supper?" the waitress asks. She is wearing a black dress under a white apron.

"A cheese sandwich and orange juice now," I decide, now that I've broken Passover. *If G-d wants me to do things to please him, he really shouldn't be trying to kill me*, I think.

"And for supper?" She scribbles down my sandwich in her notebook.

"A cheese and mushroom omelette and apple juice," I say. It's a shame they don't have Diet Coke on the menu.

"Any pudding?" I shake my head, pulling the covers up, rolling onto my front, untangling myself from the tubes.

"I'll see you later," the pantry waitress says.

I fall asleep immediately. When I wake up I phone my parents.

"Hello," Mum says, answering my call. "How are you, precious?"

"I'm hooked up to a bag of blood. Just been sleeping," I say.

"I wish we could visit you," Mum says, sounding upset.

"Me too," I say. "They're looking after me really well in here."

"I'm glad to hear it," Mum says. "Speak to you later, darling."

"Yes, of course," I say. "How's my Fluffy?"

"He's just had his second lunch and I've put him outside in the garden."

"Does he miss me?" I ask.

"He keeps sitting outside your bedroom door, wondering where you are. Sweet Fluffball."

"Tell him I'll be home soon."

"I will, darling," Mum says.

"Bye," I say.

Eventually, my bag of blood is empty.

At about five o'clock Dr Goldberg comes to see me. "We're going to give you another platelet transfusion," he says.

"OK," I say. "Where are you from?"

"South Africa, Johannesburg," he says.

"I like your accent," I say.

"That's very kind of you," he says. "Platelets are on their way." Pulling the door shut behind him, he goes out.

I find a Miss Marple to watch on ITV3 – *Towards Zero*, one of my favourites. I can keep my eyes open now, I discover.

A nurse brings the bag of platelets. I still find it strange that they are yellow.

"Hi, I'm Shula, I'm your nurse for today."

"Hello, Shula," I say, my mind blank from my low haemoglobin and platelets.

She washes some saline through my port then connects it to the tube coming out of the bag of platelets. The yellow liquid starts to run into my port and then into my body. After the platelet transfusion comes the next bag of blood. Watching the red liquid run into my body I feel much better already.

I fall asleep at 9 o'clock, after doing my body scan meditation. When I wake up, it's morning and the start of a new day. Opening my curtains I can see the weak sunshine in the car park, and in the distance, a beautiful copper beech tree.

Chapter 52

"Your blood results are much better," Dr Goldstein says two days later, after one more blood transfusion and one more platelet transfusion. "There's a bank holiday tomorrow, so you can go home today."

I certainly feel much better.

"Thank you for making me better," I say. "I'll call Mum now."

"I'll see you next week for a follow-up appointment," he says. "Your haemoglobin is now ninety-two and your platelets are twenty-five, still below what they should be but better than they were."

It's Thursday now, about 11 o'clock in the morning. I call home.

"Mum, you can come and pick me up," I say when she answers the phone.

"Already, sweetie? What about your discharge letter?"

"They'll post it," I say. "They want to get me home before the bank holiday."

"I'll be there in half an hour," Mum says.

Back home, I see my darling brother who's here for two weeks from Abroad. It's good to see him, but over the next ten days I'm in bed most of the time: I'm so weak after my treatment. I'm collapsed in bed when there's a knock at my door.

"Come in," I say.

"I can't, I have to stay here," Carl says, opening the door. I can see his sweet face. He's come from Israel and has had both shots of the vaccine but is still required to quarantine. During the course of his two-week trip he has to take six Covid tests.

"How are you feeling?" he asks, his hazel eyes full of concern.

"Happy to see you," I say, smiling at him. "Sad we can't have a hug. Wiped out."

"You're having a terrible time," he says. "I'm glad I'm here to look after you lot. Are you going to make it up for supper?"

"Yes," I say. "Can you send Mum here, please, I need a bath."

"Sure," he says, "I'm just going to get on with some reading."

My brother always has so much work to do.

"See you in a bit," I say.

"See you at supper," he says. I hear his footsteps retreat. Sitting up in bed I check my two horoscope apps: Sanctuary and Nebula. Sanctuary says it's a good day for romance, which makes me chuckle. Nebula recommends starting a work project with others. The astrological apps don't seem to realise the country is in lockdown.

"Here I am, sweetie," Mum says. "Your brother says you'd like a bath."

"Yes please,".

Mum goes into the bathroom, turns on the taps, and I can hear the water running. Hauling myself out of bed, I pick up my bright pink Marks and Spencer dressing gown with marshmallow pink hearts and follow Mum into the bathroom.

Mum sits on the laundry bin. I take my clothes off and lower myself into the bath. An apricot paw comes round the door.

"Hi Fluffy," I say. He climbs the three stairs and sits next to Mum. Sitting in the bath, I spider my fingers along the edge. He jumps up, trying to catch my fingers. He leaps onto the edge of the bath, where he used to sit as a kitten.

"Come down, Fluffball," Mum says, as the six kilogram cat teeters on the edge of the bath. He jumps down and then settles behind the laundry bin, by the radiator.

"How are you feeling, darling?" Mum asks

"Tired," I say, "Very tired."

"It's your platelets and haemoglobin, they're still much too low," Mum says. She's been sitting on the laundry basket while I have my bath all my life up 'til when I was about ten, and then this last year of lockdown. I am prone to feeling dizzy and sick in the bath now, and don't like to be in here on my own in case I drown.

"I'm so glad my brother's here," I say, opening my eyes, watching the bubbles rise over the front of my body. I have sensitive skin and have to use Sanex hypoallergenic bubble bath as anything else irritates my skin and gives me thrush. I have had thrush A LOT on chemo, caused by low white blood count, I suppose.

"It's so good to have my boy here," Mum says.

"It's not fair that I'm so ill I can barely speak to him," I say, holding back the tears. They break through anyway and cascade down my cheeks.

"Don't cry, darling," Mum strokes my tiny amount of soft, fuzzy baby hair. "You'll get better and …"

"Can we go back to the flat for a couple of days?" I ask. "I haven't been to my flat since my brother was last here in October and it's now April."

"Let's aim for that then," Mum says.

I turn over onto my front and the bubbles close over my bottom and shoulders.

"You never regret having a bath, do you," I say. "It's always worth doing."

"Let's get you out now," Mum says, holding out my towel. I step into it, and she wraps it around me and then picks my pale blue La Senza towelling robe from the hook above the laundry bin, and I put it on.

"Come on Fluffball," Mum says, but he doesn't move. She moves the laundry bin away from the wall and pulls him out. We exit the bathroom.

Back at the flat – it feels good to be here. I do really love my flat. It's so quiet and peaceful. My brother works in his room and when he has breaks he cooks meals for us and we watch series three of the top Israeli show *Shtisel* about the goings on in a religious community in Jerusalem. The hero, Akiva, is played by the heart-throb Michael Aloni, and *oh my*. It's an eventful series, covering death, pregnancy, child removal by social services, broken engagements, a religious woman taking secret driving lessons and Akiva's career as a painter.

"We've done jolly well to watch the whole series," my brother says, as we sit down to our last lunch together before our parents collect us in the evening.

"Yes, thank you so much for being here," I say, putting my arm around him, which I'm finally allowed to do now his twelve days of quarantine are over.

"I'll come back soon," he says. I can feel myself crying again. Must not make brother feel guilty for having a life.

"I miss you so much when you're not here," I say. "Lockdown has been terrible." My tears flow.

"Well, soon you'll have your second vaccination and you can visit me," he says, patting my shoulder.

"Yes," I say, pretty sure I won't be well enough to go on a plane anytime soon.

Palliative Chemo Side Effects

- Vaginal dryness and vaginismus. It just doesn't get wet down there at all and the vagina won't expand. So, if you want to do sexuals whilst having chemo, forget it. There's a topical oestrogen cream that I tried but it didn't make a lot of difference. See also: Astroglide, Skyn, KY Jelly, Vaseline, butter (probably), Durex play gels and so on.

- Loss of libido. Due to the above but also a mental change. Is this a menopause thing? I'm not sure.

- Dry mouth. I have Glandosane synthetic saliva to spray into my mouth, lemon flavour. I also use a special toothpaste, Duraphat 2800, and a soft brush so I don't hurt my gums, both from my dentist.

- Hair loss. On this chemo – GemCarbo – hair grows but then falls out. I have some hair on my head but every morning I wake up to a hair-covered pillow. It looks like £21.99 acrylic wigs from Amazon for the rest of my life. Acrylic hair loses its shine and develops dreadlocks and knots. Just running my hand through my fake hair, I encounter knots and have to pull the strands of hair apart to remove them.

- On the plus side, very little hair on legs, underarms, forearms and bikini line.

- Eyebrow thinning. I use a Nars brow pencil and no longer pluck my eyebrows at all.

- Weaker fingernails and toenails. I don't have Pro Gel or shellac fingernails anymore, but still have Pro Gel toenails. At the moment they're fluorescent pink with a top layer of glitter called Shining Armour. Painted toenails make me feel so much better in the summer.

- Difficulties and pain whilst swallowing. This is called oesophagitis and is caused by chemo. Omeprazole twice daily relieves it.

- Dry skin on hands. My hands are crocodile-scaled. I hate hand cream but if you don't, Aveeno is the one my nurses recommend.

- Fatigue. I have to sleep in the afternoon and still go to bed at nine o'clock at night, waking between five and five thirty in the morning.
- Weight loss. At the start of my chemo journey I put on half a stone during nine cycles and another half stone during radiotherapy which wiped me out. And a stone from drinking. Now, however, my size eight clothes hang off me. On the plus side, my fake boobs stand up on their own and I can wear backless and strappy tops. I used to be a 28FF, but now I'm probably a D or DD. I prefer my silicone chest as I no longer live under the tyranny of the underwired bra. I even have a yellow Matthew Williamson triangle bikini top!
- Constant nausea. I take cyclizine at mealtimes and ondansetron between meals, twice per day. This is much better than puking up all my food.
- Constipation, which is exacerbated by the fifty mg of morphine I take each day. What helps: Laxido sachets twice a day, flaxseed, senna, sodium docusate. But these remedies don't always work, and I often find Pilates or personal training gets things moving.
- Diarrhoea. Just after my last chemo I had this for three days. Better out than in but there are drugs to help such as loperamide.
- Lowered platelet count. Platelets are important because they make the blood clot. After the last chemo my platelets crashed, and when I was really ill a few weeks ago, they went down to two. Three platelet transfusions brought the count up to twenty-five, which is still much too low.
- Lowered haemoglobin. This should be at around one hundred and fifty, but mine went down to fifty-three, which explains why I was so exhausted. I had three blood transfusions in hospital, to bring the count up to ninety-two.

- Itchy scalp where new hair is trying to grow through. I use Neutrogena T-gel shampoo.
- Interestingly, I think GemCarbo has a positive effect on my mood. My last depression, after Fluffball went missing, was out of sequence as my mood had just been up for about ten weeks rather than the usual five months. My mood dropped to around four on the bipolar mood scale, where five is a normal mood. The panther didn't appear but I couldn't look at my tarot cards for six months. This was my longest depression ever, but also the mildest. I came out of it in mid-March and my mood is cheerful and positive but not so high that I can't read or write. My focus on writing, tarot and astrology goes into a flow state, which is unusual for me as often when hypomanic I can't keep still or focus. I wonder whether other bipolar people on GemCarbo or similar have noticed this? More research is needed.
- Unfortunately, I'm still buying a lot of stuff I don't need from Amazon, although I am now managing to save up to publish this book before I die.
- A constant cold due to weakened immune system. I've had this cold for years.
- Itching all over body. Aloe vera helps soothe it. The radiotherapy I've just had to try to reduce back pain made my back insanely itchy for two weeks. And, so far, hasn't helped the pain at all.
- Thrush, due to weakened immune system.

Chapter 53

MAY 2021

"Now, lie very still," the radiotherapy nurse says. "Put your hands down by your sides."

"My feet are cold," I say. I'm lying on a hard platform, on my back, with my feet exposed.

I'm having radiotherapy because my oncologist thinks it may help to ease the terrible pain in my upper back caused by the cancer.

"Better?" the nurse asks, putting a blanket on my chest which reaches down to my feet.

"Yes, thank you," I say. "My knees are uncomfortable,"

"Ok, we'll move the pillow up a bit," she says. "No, don't move, we'll do it." There are two of them as I lie on my back staring at the ceiling. One moves the knee support and I stretch my legs over it.

"Yes, that's better," I say, feeling more comfortable.

"Now, just lie as still as possible," the blonde one says.

"OK," I say.

They leave the room. The machine closes over me, the jaws of a sabre-toothed tiger.

I keep my eyes open, close them as the whirring starts.

"Now hold your breath," a disembodied voice says. They must be in the Perspex box.

"Breathe away," I sigh my breath out.

"Now we're going to start the machine," she says. I think it's the brunette.

The machine whirrs and clicks. I keep my eyes closed. It travels up and down my body.

"All done," a voice says. "Stay as still as possible, we're coming to get you out."

A few minutes later, they open the machine.

"Is that it?" I ask, when I can see the two nurses again.

"Yes, that's it," the blonde one says. "The actual treatment is only five minutes. What takes the time is getting you into position."

"Oh, I see," I say, moving a leg.

"No, stay still," the brunette says. "We need to lower the platform before you get down."

The machine whirrs as the platform drops.

"OK, you can sit up now," the blonde says.

Sitting up, I take off the hospital gown and put my vest top back on. Moving over to the chair, I untie my shoelaces and slip my feet into my orange trainers.

"My glasses," I say, and the blonde hands them to me.

"Thank you," I say. "Are there any side effects I should be looking out for?"

"Your back will feel itchy for a few days," the brunette says. "Put some E45 cream on it."

"OK, thank you," I walk to the car where Mum is waiting. Although she's my carer, she's not allowed in due to Covid restrictions.

"How was it, darling?"

"Fine, I say. "The actual treatment took only five minutes, setting up the machine took most of the time. We need to get some E45 cream as my back will be sore."

"Is it going to be all blistered and burnt like last time?" Mum asks, no doubt remembering the severe burns I suffered from two previous radiotherapy treatments.

"No, I don't think so, not from just one five-minute treatment." I say, as we set off home via the pharmacy to purchase the E45 cream.

It hurts. It's prickly heat beneath my skin. The E45 doesn't seem to help so we alternate it with Aloe Vera. The pain goes on for two weeks.

"Right, so this is the reduced dose," Luisa says to me as she makes me a bed at chemo: chair backrest down, legs up, sheet then pillow and blanket.

Slipping off my wig and my trousers, I slide under the blanket. First, I have the port flushed with saline, then an anti-sickness drug through the drip, and I take an anti-sickness pill. Next gemcitabine for about forty minutes, loo break, then carboplatin for about forty minutes.

Ten minutes before the end of the carboplatin I call Dad and ask him to pick me up. I pull on my wig and trousers and two sweaters – it's still cold in early May. Saying goodbye to the nurses, I make my way down the steps and see Dad outside in the silver Mercedes.

"How was it?" Dad asks.

"Fine," I say, looking out for the rabbits as we drive past. Two of them are feeding by the hedge.

"Look, bunnies," I say.

Back at home, I'm fine on Tuesday night but vomiting by Wednesday lunchtime after my barre class.

Mum rings the cancer hospital.

"Take her to A & E," Luisa says.

"We're not going there, they can't access her port," Mum says.

By Wednesday night I have a temperature and Mum gives me paracetamol.

"Perhaps I'm not recovered from the radiotherapy," I say, after vomiting again.

"You shouldn't have had chemo whilst you're so weak," Mum says, stroking the tufty baby hair on my head.

"Or we should have refused it," I say.

I'm ill for a few more days. My temperature comes down, but I can't swallow without a terrible pain in my chest, even when trying to drink a glass of water.

"That's oesophagitis," my oncologist says when he calls. "Let's put the omeprazole up to two a day and see what happens." I take cyclizine at mealtimes, with ondansetron between meals.

The pain in my oesophagus goes. I've been off omeprazole during the five weeks off chemo and the new double dose works well. I can swallow, and my temperature comes down. I move my suppertime to four thirty in the afternoon and this stops the vomiting at night.

I start having five small meals every day: breakfast at seven, mid-morning snack at about ten thirty, lunch at twelve to twelve thirty. Then I sleep for an hour or two. When I wake up, I have fruit and ice cream and then a very light supper of cottage cheese on toast or half a baked potato with steamed broccoli, by five at the latest. The night-time sickness stops.

I have a couple of weeks off chemo to recover but I am starting it again on May twenty-fifth on an even lower dose. Let's hope it works and the cancer doesn't make it to my skull and brain.

Meanwhile, we seem to be keeping Spitfire's hay fever in abeyance. He has half a steroid tablet every other day and half a Piriton every day. His eyes have stopped streaming and he has stopped scratching his face, so it must not be itchy anymore. Poor Precious Angel Fluffball.

He has taken to lying on my bed when I don't feel well. He's so amazing, he just curls up on my bed and sleeps while I sit in my chair to write. It's so comforting and restful to watch him sleep. Sometimes he climbs up on the windowsill and gazes out: looking for his enemy, the cat next door, or just keeping an eye on his territory. He is my life, my life-saving kitten. Just being with him is all I need as I embark on this stage of life. I'm forty-two now, my birthday was last week on the fifteenth May.

My friends come round for caterpillar birthday cake. My new friend Monica from barre, then Hannah, then Ben and Geoff. As I enter my forty-third year I am at peace with my circumstances, life and the world. We're coming out of lockdown and I've been to the Destiny shop at the farm and, with Mum, to the farm shop, the greengrocer and the garden centre. My life begins to expand again.

How to Look Stylish During Chemotherapy

- There are make-up classes for people with breast cancer. I haven't been to one, but I heard of them about eight years ago. Your skin may become more sensitive, and they will help you.
- How to draw on eyebrows: I have an excellent eyebrow pencil with which I fill in the gaps in my brows. Seven or eight years ago, when I had no eyebrows, I drew them on with a blue/green glitter eyeliner. Pencil then glitter is probably the best way to do it.
- Buy stick-on eyelashes. They come in strips and are easy to put on. I investigated individual lash treatments, but they need at least some of your lashes to bond to, so they were not suitable for me.
- Blusher puts a bit of colour into your cheeks.
- Get a good eyebrow pencil for bottom lids.
- And a good liquid eyeliner for cats' eyes on upper lids.
- Lipstick – something hydrating as lips will be dry from chemo.
- Lip balm under your lipstick or a tinted lip balm instead of lipstick.

- A light foundation if you need it. Anything too heavy will clog your pores and may aggravate your skin.
- Mascara: you won't need this on your false lashes but if you're where I am, on chemotherapy which doesn't take all your hair, use mascara.
- Concealer.
- Check Cruelty-Free Kitty to see which brands are cruelty-free. Garnier now is, which is great, but many of the cheaper brands are not.
- For lighter coverage than foundation, get a BB cream.
- Get a fun make-up bag. I have a gorgeous new one which is velvet with giraffes on a velvet background, made by my friend. It is wipe clean inside.
- Back in 2013 when I first had chemo, I was given a wig by the NHS. It was worth about £120 and, when it fell to pieces, I bought bright, cheerful acrylic ones. I have nine now in pink, peacock blue, purple, burgundy, bright red, orange, black with red streaks, brown and light brown with ash blonde and purple highlights. Get a few different ones. They come with wig liners, and you can buy stands on Amazon. If you don't want to wear a wig, there are hats with hair sticking out at the bottom, or turbans or scarves. You really can pay any amount of money for a wig. Human hair ones cost hundreds of pounds, but I wouldn't recommend them as they have to be washed with shampoo. Also, I wouldn't be comfortable wearing someone else's hair. There are some good, more expensive acrylic wigs available: shop around.
- You may change the way you dress. At the start I wore high-necked dresses to hide my scars, but now my chest has healed I wear low-cut tops. No need for a bra anymore and as a former 28FF it is so liberating just to throw a vest top or strappy dress

on. Also, I save a fortune on bras. Wear what you want. Other people won't judge your scars: the problem is in your head. I wear backless dresses despite a huge scar across my back from TRAM flap surgery.

- If you've lost or put on a lot of weight from chemo, ask your Macmillan nurse about the one-off grant of £200-300 to help you buy clothes in your new size. It is not means-tested.
- Smile if you possibly can. It will make you look and feel better.
- Just do what you want, wear what you want, don't wear make-up or a wig if you don't want to. It's up to you.

What to Eat When You Have No Appetite

- Scones with cream cheese, lemon curd or marmalade.
- Mango, melon or pineapple with ice cream.
- Cheesecake, chocolate cake.
- Stewed or baked apples.
- Toast with Marmite and cream cheese.
- Half a baked potato with cottage cheese.
- Steamed broccoli.
- Salad.
- Sliced apple or pear.
- Toast with pesto and goats' cheese.
- Protein drinks, there are many different ones available.
- Apple, pear or orange juice.
- Biscuits. I like oat wholemeal ones.
- Muesli. I like the ones with tropical fruit and I add milk and honey.

These foods have become my staple diet since becoming nauseated on chemo. You may find completely different foods suit your stomach.

Chapter 54

We're sitting in the garden of Pizza Express in Radlett. I'm out with my barre and Pilates crew to celebrate my birthday. It's the seventeenth of May so we're also celebrating the beginning of the end of lockdown.

"I saw there's an offer," Honey says. She has a huge mane of blonde, curly hair, a lion's mane. "A bottle of Peroni with your meal for free."

"It's a small Peroni, small glass of wine or a soft drink," the waiter says. I recognise him of course because I've been coming to this restaurant for most of my life and it seems he has always been here.

"Glass of Pinot Grigio," Honey says. "Miriam will have one as well, won't you?"

"Oh, go on then," Miriam says, smiling. She's tall, slim and tanned with short brown and blonde streaked hair. Honey and Miriam have been best friends for years.

"I'll have a Diet Coke please," I say. "One slice of lime."

"And for you?" he asks Anna who is sitting at the far end of the table.

"I'll just have tap water."

"We made it through lockdown," Miriam says. "Well done us."

I look around the table at my three friends. Two – Rebecca and Elena aren't here yet, but after many years, I finally have a group of girlfriends again. We see each other online at least three times a week.

"Phone call for you," the waiter says, rushing out.

"It's me," Elena says. "I'm so sorry, I was all set to be on time but there's terrible traffic on the motorway."

"Don't worry," I say. "We're sitting in the sunshine about to have a drink, we'll see you soon."

"Elena?" Honey asks, I nod.

"She's running late," I say.

"Why doesn't that surprise me?" Honey asks. "She manages to be late for barre. How can you be late for a Zoom meeting?"

We all laugh at the foible of our friend who is, indeed, always late. We all love her: she's the kindest, sweetest, funniest person but she is always late.

"Wow, I love your trousers," I say to Honey, who is wearing black PVC trousers.

"They're really good," she says. "So comfortable, look," she shows me the elasticated waistband.

"I just love them," I say

Miri and Anna are talking to each other down the other end of the table.

"And I love your hair," I say to Honey. "Have you had it coloured?" Her hair is bleached very blonde.

"I washed it yesterday," she says, "that's all."

"It looks fab," I say.

"Thank you, darling," she says, and sips her Pinot Grigio, which has just arrived.

"This is lovely," Miriam says, "I've been looking forward to today for ages."

"Me too," I say, and I have. It's only my second meal out since lockdown ended.

"Sorry, sorry, sorry." Rebecca says, arriving at the table weighed down by two bags of what I hope are presents for me. She takes a couple of white balloons out of one bag, already inflated. "Have a special birthday," the balloons say in gold writing.

"Becca," Miriam says, "It's so great to see you in real life."

We all have hugs, which we're allowed to do from today, the end of phase one of lifting the lockdown restrictions. I have a long hug with Miri, and it feels so good we don't want to stop hugging.

"I haven't hugged anyone except my parents for ages," I say. "Well, I hugged my brother a few times when he was here recently, but this is the first hug with someone to whom I'm not related for about fourteen months."

We go round the table hugging each other.

"Nothing beats a hug," Anna says.

"I was so excited teaching barre this morning," Becca says. "I just wanted to get through the class and get ready to meet you all." Becca looks amazing in her leopard print coat and long dark brown hair with highlights.

"It's amazing to see you all," I say as it starts pouring and we move across at speed to the table under the big umbrella.

"Yes, it is," Anna says.

"You should come to Becca's online classes," I say, settling down at the new table .

"Oh look, she's here, hi Elena," Miriam says as Elena comes through the door wearing a glamorous black double denim outfit with black knee-high boots.

"So sorry I'm late girls," she says, dumping her bag on the chair next to mine. "Terrible traffic on the motorway."

"Well, you're here now," Becca says, giving her a hug.

"I just wanted to say," I say, as the six of us sit at our table, rain pouring down. "It's been a long time since I've had a group of girlfriends, so thank you all for being my friends."

"We have a special bond, all of us," Elena says. "Friendships built over lockdown are the most special friendships. So, thank you all for coming to my classes and…"

"Thank you for running the classes," Honey says. "They've been a life saver."

"For me too," Becca says, smiling.

Elena dispenses umbrella hats and we all put them on for a photo.

"These are amazing," I say, pulling the headband down around my purple wig. We all look at each other with our rainbow umbrella hats on and we burst out laughing. I love my girls.

"I was wondering," I say, after the waiter has taken our orders and a few photos, some with and some without our umbrella hats. "Could we please open my presents now?"

"Yes, let's do it," Becca says, handing me two huge bags. The first thing is the Witches' Tarot.

"Oh, I really wanted this," I say, "thank you so much everyone."

"I know, it does rather take away from the surprise," Becca says.

The next one is soft, and they're all wrapped in leopard print paper. Opening it, I see it's the metallic silver Nike sports bra Becca has, and I asked for. "It's so silver and shiny, I love it." It will look great under dresses.

"Now it's the main present," I say. Opening it, my jaw drops in amazement. It's even more stunning than it looked on the internet: a dodecahedron – the twelve-point infinity star.

"I'm going to wrap him up very carefully," I say, wrapping him in the Nike bra.

"Stacie says she cleansed it for you," Becca says.

"She's lovely," Anna says. "I just bought a couple of crystals from her, and she spent so much time talking to me about them."

"Yes, she is very kind," Becca says.

"What do you do with it?" Elena asks.

"Meditate, I guess," I say. "I'll message Stacie later." She's my crystal dealer, I've bought several crystals from her and she has become a new lockdown friend too.

There's still one more thing in the bag: it's a beautiful light-up vase of purple and pink fake roses.

"Oh, I adore it," I say.

"I know you like pink and purple," Becca says.

"I love all my presents, thank you everyone." We sit at our table, eating, drinking and chatting until about a quarter to three. The sun comes out again and we all move to stand in it.

"Thank you for the best birthday." I say.

Epilogue

A nd so, after all that came before, I've found happiness. It's being with my cat, my family and my friends. It's writing and tarot and astrology. Happiness doesn't come from outside: from achievements or having a boyfriend. Instead, it's spending time studying what I love; getting paid for my work as a tarot reader which I enjoy so much. It's reading a good book, watching my garden birds, writing when I wake up. I am content with my life, grateful for it.

I am very lucky to be able to extract joy from my simple tastes and to be so easily pleased. Watching a new bullfinch in the garden, Spitfire lying on my bed whilst I write, watching tennis with Mum – all fulfil me.

Well done me!